EveryWoman's®
Beauty
Basics

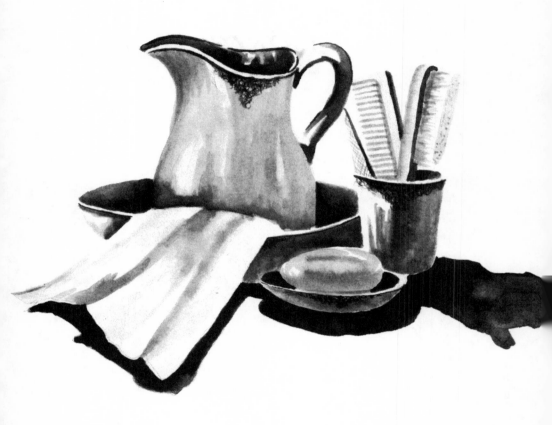

EveryWoman's®

Beauty

Basics

The Guide to Healthy Skin, Hair, and Nails

by Laura Flynn McCarthy

Illustrations by Claire Moritz

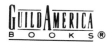

GUILDAMERICA BOOKS®

Doubleday Book & Music Clubs, Inc.   Garden City, New York

Book design by Robert Aulicino
Art direction by Diana Klemin

For my mother, Elizabeth Flynn,
who taught me the basics way back when.

Contents

Foreword

Recently you've noticed your hair is thinning. Your doctor says it could be hormonal and suggests some blood tests. Your stylist says it could be mechanical damage and suggests a new haircut. The label on the "hair thickener" in your drugstore claims that using the product will make your hair look more voluminous.

Whom do you believe? Whom can you really trust when it comes to advice about skin, hair, and nails? All of these sources may be correct in some ways, but all of them have their biases. Have a professional facial and your "esthetician" may say you should *never* wash with soap; the next day your dermatologist may *recommend* a particular soap; and in your drugstore there may be five soaps that claim to be appropriate for your skin type.

This book is designed to help you cut through all the advice to find the answers that are right for you. The information herein results from interviews with the nation's most respected dermatologists; most sought-after stylists, nail technicians, and facialists; and most knowledgeable scientists on the research and development staffs of the country's top cosmetic companies. It is a book that will tell you the truth about the way to care for your skin, hair, and nails, as well as dispel the myths. It may even save you some money by preventing you from buying products you don't need.

After you've heard all the cosmetic claims, read all the new studies, and tried the latest products, one fact becomes clear: taking good care of yourself means using common sense, which is why this book takes a no-nonsense approach to skin, hair, and nail care. When you make the right decisions about caring for your skin, hair, and nails, the result is not only something that you will feel but a change that everyone you encounter will see.

This book was put together with the invaluable support and assistance of the following people who generously offered their time, expertise, and wisdom. My heartfelt thanks to you all: Richard K. Scher, M.D., Professor of Dermatology and head of the nail section at Columbia Presbyterian Medical Center; C. Ralph Daniel, M.D., Clinical Professor of Medicine (Dermatology) at the University of Mississippi Medical Center, Jackson; John H. Epstein, M.D., Clinical Professor of Dermatology at the University of California in San Francisco; Darrell Rigel, M.D., Associate Professor of Dermatology at New York University Medical School; Jack L. Lesher, Jr., M.D., Associate Professor of Dermatology at the Medical College of Georgia in Augusta; Peter J. Lynch, M.D., Professor and Head of the Department of Dermatology at the University of Minnesota in Minneapolis; Denise Jacob at the American Academy of Dermatology; Joyce Ayoub at the Skin Cancer Foundation; the folks at the National Psoriasis Foundation; Sheila Hoar Zahm, Sc.D., epidemiologist at the National Cancer Institute; John Corbett, Ph.D., Vice President of Scientific and Technical Affairs, Clairol; David Cannell, Ph.D., Corporate Vice President of Technology, Redken Laboratories; Beth Minardi, color director of Minardi Minardi Salon in New York City; Amy Paller, M.D., Associate Professor of Pediatrics and Dermatology at Northwestern University Medical School; Jean Bolognia, M.D., Associate Professor of Dermatology, Yale Medical School; Marianne O'Donoghue, M.D., Associate Professor of Dermatology at Rush-Presbyterian/St. Luke's Medical School in Chicago; and the folks in the press office at the Food and Drug Administration.

Many thanks, also, to my editor, Barbara Greenman, for her patience and guidance.

I extend very special thanks to my family—the Flynns and the McCarthys—for their unfailing support.

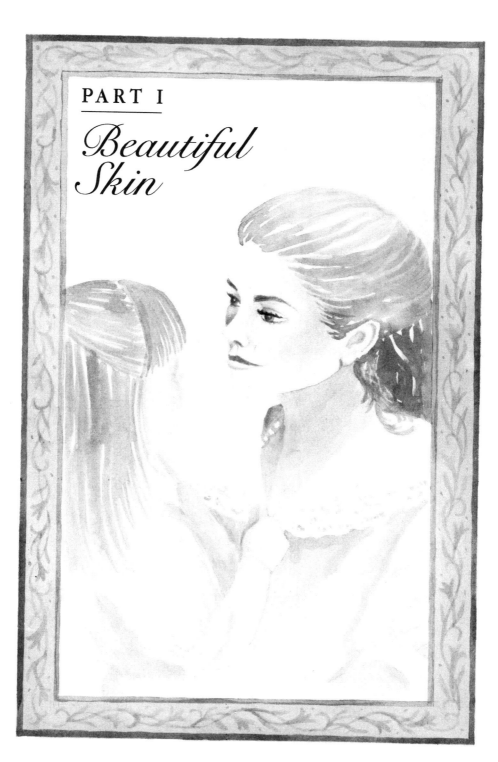

PART I

Beautiful Skin

CHAPTER 1

The Five Ages of Your Skin

Your skin is the largest organ of your body, and it has the remarkable function of protecting every other organ and part inside you. It is also the means by which your body regulates its temperature. Your skin is your natural barrier against the outside world, and it is integral to the way the outside world perceives you. Get a stomach cramp, a headache, or a kidney stone, and no one has to know about it but you. But break out in a rash, and the whole world knows. No wonder, then, that skin not only can trigger emotional responses within us but is also affected by them and is a reflection of them. And no wonder that beautiful skin—with imperceptible pores, a uniform color, and a certain translucence—is considered one of the greatest physical assets one can have.

What is the secret to beautiful skin? Don't let the advertisements fool you. It has nothing to do with using any one moisturizer or makeup or soap. It has to do with your total lifestyle. Of course, having parents with flawless skin can help; certain qualities of the skin do tend to be inherited. But even if you don't have the genes of a supermodel, you can make your skin look its best by being sensible about the way you live: eating well, getting enough exercise and enough sleep, avoiding too much sun exposure, keeping stress to a minimum, not smoking, not drinking alcohol to excess, and not going overboard on facial cleansing are all elements of a great complexion. And seeing a dermatologist for help when skin problems do arise is important. Understanding just how

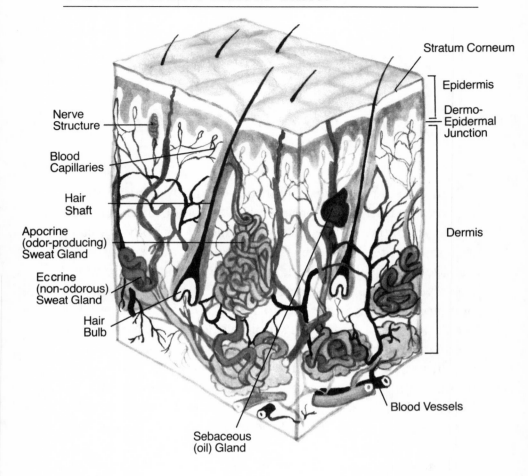

Stratum Corneum

Epidermis

Dermo-
Epidermal
Junction

Nerve
Structure

Blood
Capillaries

Hair
Shaft

Apocrine
(odor-producing)
Sweat Gland

Dermis

Eccrine
(non-odorous)
Sweat Gland

Hair
Bulb

Blood Vessels

Sebaceous
(oil) Gland

your skin functions is also basic to knowing how to care for it. Here is a small course in what your skin looks like from the inside out.

The Anatomy of Skin

Your skin has two primary layers: the epidermis, or upper portion, which includes the surface, and the dermis, or lower portion just below the epidermis, which houses the blood vessels, nerve fibers, and sweat and oil glands. Between these two layers lies an undulating line of cells known as the dermo-epidermal junction. Below the dermis lies a layer of fat known as the subcutis, which, like a boxspring to a mattress, gives the skin flexibility and resilience. Both the epidermis and the dermis comprise dozens of smaller layers, all of which help to carry out the normal functions of your skin.

The Epidermis

If the subcutis were the boxspring, and the dermis were the mattress, then the epidermis would qualify as the bottom sheet on the mattress. Even though your epidermis is only about as thick as a piece of paper, it contains as many as twenty different layers. The cells of your epidermis renew themselves an average of every twenty-eight days. New cells are constantly being produced in the bottom layer of the epidermis known as the basal cell layer. Those cells then migrate over the next two weeks to the top layer of your skin, called the stratum corneum. On the way up to the skin surface, the basal cells become squamous cells, which make up the thickest layer in the middle of the epidermis. Once at the skin surface, skin cells remain in the stratum corneum for about another two weeks, until they are shed. Your skin is shedding, usually imperceptibly, a little bit everyday. Anyone who has ever had to wear a plaster cast has seen the buildup of shedded skin cells over several weeks. Sun damage in the form of sunburn can also make the shedding perceptible by speeding up the rate at which those upper layers are shed, resulting in what many women refer to as peeling skin.

The basal layer of your skin is also home to your skin's pigment cells, the melanocytes. These cells produce the pigment melanin, which gives your skin its usual color as well as the darker color you achieve when you get a suntan. Black and other dark-skinned individuals actually have the same number of pigment cells as light-skinned people, but those cells tend to be larger and produce a greater amount of pigment, giving dark skin a more uniform darker tone.

When you look in the mirror, you see the stratum corneum layer of your skin, the uppermost layer of the epidermis. It is composed of dead cells that contain the protein keratin, the same protein that is found in your hair and fingernails. This layer is sometimes referred to as the horny layer because the tightly compacted keratin is similar to the dense keratin of the horns of such animals as the rhinoceros. The stratum corneum layer of your skin is sometimes also called the barrier layer because it provides a waterproof barrier between the outside world and the dermis layer of your skin— preventing too much water from either getting in or evaporating from the surface. It is also a barrier against potentially harmful elements in the environment such as pollutants, cigarette smoke, and sunlight.

Consider the structure of the stratum corneum the next time you choose a skin cream or lotion. Be suspicious of any product that carries claims of "nourishing" the skin or providing the collagen or vitamins that "skin loses with age." First of all, cosmetics, by law, cannot penetrate below the stratum corneum layer of the skin; any substance that does is classified as a drug. Secondly, nothing can "nourish" the stratum corneum because it is composed of dead cells that obviously cannot eat. Finally, exotic ingredients such as collagen and placental extracts may sound as though they can restore a youthful glow to skin, but remember that their molecular weights are inevitably too great for them to penetrate below the stratum corneum. These ingredients are rarely, if ever, worth the extra money that they add to the cost of a product. (For more on choosing skin care products, see Chapter 6, pages 90–105.)

The Dermis

The dermis, in a sense, is the heart of your skin. It houses your skin's blood vessels, nerves, sweat glands, sebaceous (oil) glands, and the roots of your hair follicles. It also gives flexibility and strength to the skin by virtue of its elastin and collagen fibers. These are the resilient fibers that enable your skin to bounce back after it has been stretched. The gradual depletion and stretching of these fibers with age and sun exposure is what causes skin to sag and gives it a less youthful appearance.

Anytime blood appears on the surface of your skin, whether through an injury or by squeezing of a blemish, you have reached the dermis layer of the skin and you run the risk of causing a scar. Superficial injuries to the skin that affect only the epidermis do not result in scars. It is for this reason that doctors warn against aggressive treatment of the skin.

The "Skin Type" Myth

Any woman who has ever picked up a beauty magazine is familiar with the notion of skin type. Not to be confused with the use of the term by dermatologists to describe a skin's susceptibility to sun damage (see Chapter 2), the cosmetic counter version of skin type classifies a woman's skin as either oily, dry, or combination (usually meaning that skin is oily on the forehead, nose, and chin—called the T-zone—and dry on the cheeks). Once her skin is labeled, a woman tends to regard it always as one of these types and looks for cosmetics that are suited to her skin.

There is some justification for following these skin types. For example, if your skin were very acne-prone, you wouldn't want to use a creamy moisturizer (probably intended for dry skin) that could potentially clog your pores. You would be better off looking for products for oily/acne-prone skin. What many women don't realize, however, is that skin type isn't constant; it can change with the seasons, with your behavior, and with your age, to name just a few factors.

For example, anyone with a sunburn has, at least temporarily, dry skin. Anyone who is skiing on a windy mountaintop needs a moisturizer because the oils on her skin are being stripped; she, too, for the time she is out on the slopes, has dry skin. On the other hand, if you work over a french fry machine at a fast food restaurant, your skin—even if it's usually dry—will be oily; it is also likely to be oily immediately after an intense exercise workout because the increased heat of your body stimulates your skin's oil glands to up oil production.

Age, too, can change your skin type. Most children, for example, have relatively dry skin. Most teenagers have oily skin, and that oil production decreases only very slowly into one's twenties, thirties, and forties. Whereas your entire T-zone may have been oily when you were twenty, by the time you're thirty just your chin may be oily and acne-prone. Many postmenopausal women have dry skin because their oil glands are not as active.

Your skin type will also vary depending on the location on your body. The skin on your face, back, and the V of your chest is likely to be much more oily than the skin on your hands, legs, and feet, which contain fewer oil glands. The skin on your feet is the thickest skin on your entire body; the skin on your eyes is the thinnest. This is one reason why you may be correct in saying you have sensitive skin if you are referring to your eyelids, but it's unlikely that you have sensitive skin on your feet.

Keeping in mind that your skin type varies and is ever-changing may help you make more realistic choices in skin care products and makeup and should enable you to have a better-equipped arsenal of cosmetics. The rest of this chapter is designed to give you a basic understanding of the types of changes you can expect to see in your skin as you age.

The Five Ages of Your Skin

Infancy

Anyone who has spent any time in a hospital nursery realizes that few infants are born with perfect skin. Most newborns have small skin blemishes of one sort or another that clear up spontaneously within a few days or may last longer or even be permanent. These include the following:

Milia. Tiny white cysts that usually occur on the nose, milia feel like tiny beads to the touch. They usually clear up on their own and should never be picked, which can cause scars.

White, dry, scaly skin. Occurring in some babies who are born several days after their due date, scaly skin is thought to be caused by a loss of the fetus's protective skin covering, the vernix caseosa. In infants who are born on time, the vernix caseosa can sometimes make the skin look greasy. Usually this covering comes off naturally with the infant's first sponge bath, but bits may remain in the folds of the skin, such as behind the ears and under the buttocks, for several days.

Rashes. About 70 percent of babies experience a rash called erythema toxicum, characterized by red blotches with small white raised centers that may even look like tiny blisters. This rash tends to occur on the face, neck, and trunk. It is most common in the first week of life and tends to go away within the next few weeks. No treatment is usually required.

Babies are also more prone to prickly heat or heat rash than adults are. Prickly heat is caused by perspiration that becomes trapped in the skin, leading to redness and inflammation of the skin. The rash resembles that of erythema toxicum, but is finer, and tends to occur in the folds of the skin, such as those around the neck and the groin. Often a prickly heat rash clears up on its own, but some parents like to apply powder or cornstarch to the area to help to keep it dry. Dressing the baby in lightweight clothing and keeping him cool in the summer can also help.

Moles. When moles are present at birth, as they are in about 1 percent of infants, they are called congenital nevi. Since these types of moles have an increased risk of developing into skin cancer than moles that develop later in life, many pediatricians like to remove them sometime during childhood. Other doctors may just watch the moles carefully to see if they undergo any changes that may signal a problem, and remove them at that time.

Hemangiomas. Vascular birthmarks, hemangiomas are red or blue lesions that consist of tiny blood vessels bunched together. They can occur anywhere on the skin, as well as in the mouth, nose, vagina, anus, or, very rarely, inside the skull or body. They can vary in size from minute to involving an entire limb. About 8 percent of infants have hemangiomas, and the cause is unknown.

Strawberry hemangiomas are soft red lesions that may or may not resemble a strawberry and are usually about one or two inches in diameter. They may be present at birth or appear during the first few months of life. Most strawberry hemangiomas grow fairly rapidly for the first six to eighteen months of life, but after a while they begin to regress in size, although they may take as long as six years to disappear completely. About 70 percent of all strawberry hemangiomas have resolved by the time children are seven years old. Of the remaining 30 percent, only those that interfere with body functions (such as lesions on the eyes, which can cause them to close) need medical treatment.

Port-wine stains. The former Soviet leader Mikhail Gorbachev probably has the most well-known example of a port-wine stain, the purplish lesion on his forehead. Red, blue, or purple vascular lesions tend to occur most commonly on the face, neck, trunk, arms, and legs and range greatly in size. They are usually flat but can become elevated as a person ages. Although they are not considered a medical concern, cosmetically they can be disabling, especially when they cover a substantial portion of the face. Because port-wine stains do not clear up spontaneously, various removal techniques have been tried over the years, including X-rays, skin grafts, dermabrasion, tattooing, and freezing the lesions with liquid nitrogen. In the last few years the removal of port-wine stains with lasers, especially the pulsed dye laser, has shown great promise. Removal with lasers has been achieved in as few as two or three office visits. The procedure can be uncomfortable and is sometimes done under local anesthesia.

Acne. In infants acne is actually quite common and is generally thought to be a reaction to maternal hormones. The acne usually occurs between four and six weeks of age and can often be "treated" simply by washing the baby's face with baby shampoo. The lesions tend to clear up within a few weeks without any treatment.

Diaper rash. Perhaps the best-known, if not indeed the most common, skin problem in infants, diaper rash on the buttocks and genitals is usually caused by leaving wet or especially soiled diapers on a baby for too long. (In contrast, rashes caused by yeast infections occur more often on the thighs, genitals, and lower abdomen but rarely on the buttocks.) Diaper rash is most common among babies who are eight to ten months old and starting to eat solid foods. It is especially likely to occur in infants who have frequent stools or diarrhea or in babies who are taking antibiotics, which can encourage the growth of yeast organisms that can infect the skin. Interestingly, diaper rash is less common in babies who are breast-fed, although no one knows why.

Diaper rash can usually be prevented by changing a baby's diaper frequently, changing it immediately after a bowel movement if possible, and not putting the diaper on so snugly that it constricts the flow of air in the area. Most diaper rashes will improve within two days with use of a cream containing zinc oxide, which provides a mechanical barrier against the wetness. Any diaper rash that doesn't clear up in three days or looks especially red and inflamed merits a consultation with your pediatrician. The rash could be a sign of another problem.

Caring for your newborn's skin should be simple if you remember that less is probably more. In most cases a sponge bath using just water and perhaps a very mild baby soap once or twice a week is enough to keep your baby looking and feeling good. Of course, infants, like all of us, should be protected from the sun. Most sunscreen manufacturers, however, don't recommend use of their products for infants under six months of age, simply because most sunscreens have not been tested for safety in this age group. Since babies may be particularly susceptible to sun damage, they should be kept in the shade whenever outside and protected with a bonnet and lightweight clothing that provides adequate coverage of all of their skin.

Childhood

Aside from the occasional skinned knee and split lip, most healthy children have few skin problems. In fact, these common injuries usually heal quickly in children because their skin cell turnover rate is slightly faster than that of adults, which accelerates the healing process. Keeping a well-stocked medicine chest, complete with bandages of varying sizes, antibacterial spray and ointment, an over-the-counter cream that contains hydrocortisone, and gauze and adhesive tape, will enable you to deal with these minor emergencies when they occur.

Another basic to a well-stocked medicine chest is a sunscreen with an SPF (sun protection factor) of 15 or higher. Studies show that most of the damage that sun does to our skin occurs before we reach age eighteen. In children signs of sun damage start early in the form of freckling, which usually begins on the nose and cheeks. While freckles may be endearing, they are really a sign that a child has had some sun damage. Freckles occur when the melanocytes of the skin deposit pigment on the skin surface, usually in an effort to provide some protection against the sun's rays. The very presence of freckles, however, is indication that the skin's pigment is not enough protection from the sun; if it were, the result would be a deep, even brown color all over the skin. Most children who freckle are fair-skinned (although even black skin can freckle). Fair-skinned children are the ones who need sunscreen protection the most. Many dermatologists recommend that applying sunscreen in the morning, particularly on fair-skinned children, should be as automatic as brushing their teeth and tying their shoes. If the sunscreen provides an SPF of 15 or higher, and your child is spending a typical day at school and outdoors (not at a beach intentionally sunning), one thorough application of sunscreen should provide enough protection for an entire day in most cases.

Parents should also make a habit of examining their children's skin. Although it's common for people to develop some distinguishing marks during childhood, such as small moles and freckles, unusually large moles or moles that grow and change noticeably over a few months should always be brought to a dermatologist's attention. In some cases such growths may indicate an increased risk of skin cancer.

Childhood is also the time when a person's allergies first assert themselves, often in the form of hives or other rashes. Hives, characterized by an itchy red rash consisting of raised red bumps with pale centers (welts), are a common allergic reaction in children and adults alike. Hives can result from allergies to foods (such as certain berries, cheeses, nuts, milk products, or shellfish), drugs (including some antibiotics and even aspirin), pollen, plants, certain skin care products, infection, bee stings, other bug bites, and many other substances.

Hives can be treated with nonprescription antihistamine tablets and with cool compresses to relieve the swelling and itching. When hives are accompanied by other symptoms such as fever or trouble swallowing and/or breathing, call your physician immediately. These may be symptoms of a more serious condition known as an anaphylactic reaction, which may require an injection of adrenaline to reduce the symptoms. Prevention of hives involves determining just what the child is allergic to (not always an easy task) and avoiding that substance in the future.

Of course, childhood is also the time for such diseases as measles, mumps, rubella (German measles), and chicken pox, all of which have, as their major symptoms, skin rashes of one sort or another. The best prevention for these conditions is following a standard schedule of vaccinations. In fact, protection from the first three conditions is available in a single injection, usually called the MMR vaccine. Your pediatrician will likely advise you about when your child needs this and other immunizations. There is also a vaccine for chicken pox available in the United States; at this writing, its use is reserved for people who would be at extremely high risk if they contracted the disease (such as people with AIDS or others who have suppressed immune systems). Many experts in the field of infectious diseases, however, predict that in the near future the use of chicken pox vaccine will become as common to pediatric practices as the MMR vaccine.

Adolescence

If you were able to film the life of your skin from the inside out, the most dramatic scenes would take place during puberty. During these years the body increases production of sex hormones, particularly the "male" hormones known as androgens that are present in both males and females. These hormones cause the sebaceous glands in the skin to enlarge, and they in turn produce more oil. At the same time the walls of the hair follicles thicken, increasing the number of cells that are shed into the follicular canal. Acne often results when those shedding cells clump together in the follicular canal, causing a blockage behind which the excess oil builds and bacteria proliferates. (For more information on the causes and treatments of acne, see Chapter 3.)

Puberty is also when many young women first notice stretch marks appearing on their skin. Stretch marks (known by the medical term *striae)* are purplish lines that eventually fade to white or silver but never completely disappear. They occur primarily on the hips, thighs, stomach, and breasts, and can arise in men as well as in women. Although no one knows what, exactly, causes stretch marks, it is thought that the surge of hormones during puberty (and also during pregnancy, when stretch marks are also common) breaks down the skin's collagen fibers, so that skin can't withstand the stress of stretching over a surface that is increasing in size as a result of extreme weight gain, normal growth of breasts and hips during puberty, or normal enlargement of the abdomen during pregnancy.

There is no proven way to prevent the formation of stretch marks, although some women swear by the daily use of moisturizers that contain cocoa butter or vitamin E on the skin. One scientific study did show that newly formed stretch marks could be eliminated through the use of retinoic acid (Retin-A); this is not an option for nursing mothers, however, because ingestion of the drug by the baby may cause problems in a newborn. Use of retinoic acid on stretch marks should be discussed with your physician. (For more on retinoic acid, see Chapter 5, pages 85–86.)

The teens are also the years of experimentation and sometimes extreme behavior, evidence of which can show up in the skin. For instance, extremely pale skin or skin that bruises easily may signal certain nutritional deficiencies and a potential eating disorder such as anorexia (self-starvation) or bulimia (the binge/purge syndrome). The teenage years are when these disorders often first arise. Yellow skin may result from consuming fad diets that emphasize too much beta carotene, a nutrient found in carrots, broccoli, and other vegetables. Sudden rashes on skin may result from reactions to new products being tried (see Chapter 4, pages 55–57, on contact dermatitis). Skin that looks exceptionally dried out may reflect overaggressive cleansing and scrubbing.

On the bright side, when well cared for, skin during the teen years can be exceptionally pretty, reflecting an active lifestyle and an energetic outlook. Keep good skin looking its best with gentle cleansing at least twice a day using lukewarm water and a mild soap or cleansing bar. Washing your hair at least once a day will prevent excess scalp oils from drifting onto facial skin, decreasing acne potential. A well-balanced diet, regular exercise, and a sensible cleansing regimen can all add up to skin that is healthy and vibrant looking.

Twenties to Forties: The Reproductive Years

After the skin upheavals of the teen years, some women feel that their skin settles down to look its best ever. Pore size begins to diminish, and the skin may become slightly drier. Women who have never had particularly oily skin may now begin to feel that they need a moisturizer to compensate for the reduced oil production in their sebaceous glands. Many women throughout their thirties and even into their forties, however, never really need a moisturizer for their skin on a daily basis.

Although acne may not go away completely (see Chapter 3), it does tend to improve in most women in this age group. Some women, however, notice increased acne flares in the week just prior to their monthly menstrual periods. This, again, probably reflects the effects of hormones on the skin.

In the first two weeks of your menstrual cycle (beginning on the day you get your period), estrogen is the dominant hormone produced in your body. Estrogen is thought to improve acne by suppressing the activity of your skin's sebaceous glands. Then, beginning at ovulation, about two weeks after the start of your period, your body increases its output of androgens and progesterone, other hormones that stimulate the sebaceous glands to produce more oil. Because it can take a week or so for a blemish to form, acne lesions tend to arise just before the start of another menstrual period and may have subsided by the time your menstrual period actually occurs. The use of antiacne medications may be particularly important during the two weeks following ovulation. Sometimes the use of oral contraceptives, which suppress the ovaries, can also help reduce premenstrual acne flares.

The skin's susceptibility to irritant reactions may also vary depending on the time of the menstrual cycle. One study from the Netherlands indicates that women are more sensitive to a common irritant called sodium lauryl sulfate at the very beginning of their menstrual cycle than at mid cycle. Although no one knows just what's behind these results, the researchers suggest that the point at which a woman is in her menstrual cycle should be considered when testing her for an irritancy to a substance.

When acne lesions that occur during the years from your twenties through your forties are accompanied by other symptoms, including excess body hair, irregular periods, and problems becoming pregnant, it is definitely time to see a doctor. These symptoms may signal an underlying hormonal imbalance, and sometimes a simple blood test can help to make a diagnosis. Once a problem is identified, your doctor may be able to prescribe treatment that can regulate your hormones and thus reduce or eliminate your symptoms.

Pregnancy and Your Skin

Few events alter one's life as much as being pregnant, and among the many changes you'll witness in your body will likely be some changes in your skin. Not every woman's skin reacts the same way to pregnancy. Some women develop the well-known "glow" of pregnancy, particularly after their first trimester, when the amount of circulating blood increases and brings a rosiness and radiance to the skin surface. Sometimes the increase in circulating blood levels can contribute to the development of spider veins or "broken blood vessels." (For more on this, see Chapter 4, pages 78–79.) Other women may experience worse acne breakouts than ever before, most likely because of hormonal surges. In some cases doctors can prescribe topical medications to treat acne flare-ups, but most are reluctant to prescribe any systemic treatment because of potentially negative effects on the developing fetus.

Many women also experience pigmentation changes in

their skin during pregnancy, especially deposits of darker pigmentation on their facial skin (a condition called melasma), and a darkening of certain areas of their body skin, such as the skin surrounding the nipples and on the genitals. (These pigmentary changes are described in more depth in Chapter 4, pages 73–77.)

About halfway through pregnancy, some women develop skin tags, tiny flaps of flesh-colored skin, on the face, neck, chest, armpits, under the breasts, or on the inner thighs. Sometimes they disappear spontaneously shortly after a woman gives birth. If they don't, they can be removed through simple excision in a brief office visit. Removal isn't necessary medically, but some women feel that they are unsightly and want them removed.

Some women also find that they bruise easily during pregnancy, especially in the last trimester. Those black and blue marks, known by the medical term *purpura,* are thought to result from the extra stress put on capillaries and the valves in your veins by the increased blood volume that your vessels are pumping during this time. Although the condition can be disconcerting, the bruising usually clears up quickly after delivery.

Fifty-Plus: Aging Skin

By age fifty most women have developed their share of "character lines" and small wrinkles and may even notice that their skin is beginning to sag. There are two different kinds of aging that your skin undergoes: photoaging (changes induced by sun exposure) and chronologic aging (changes due to normal heredity and older age).

Doctors emphasize that more than 80 percent of the symptoms we associate with aging skin are caused not by normal chronologic aging but by photoaging. Photographs of aged cloistered monks and nuns, who rarely expose their skin to the sun, offer dramatic examples of how much younger skin can look when it is protected from the sun throughout one's life. Most of us can see the same evidence by looking at the skin on our buttocks or other body part that hasn't been exposed to ultraviolet light. While some sagging of buttock skin is inevitable, there is little if any wrinkling, and skin color is likely to remain uniform, not take on the blotchy appearance of skin that has seen too much of the sun over the years.

Cigarette smoking has also been shown to increase facial wrinkling, particularly around the eyes (squint lines) and the mouth (pucker lines). Some experts believe this increased wrinkling results from the fact that nicotine constricts the blood vessels in the skin, restricting the nutrients that the blood carries to the skin's surface. Some doctors also point out that the chemicals in cigarette smoke may have direct, though currently unknown, effects on the skin. Cigarette smoking also affects the color of skin, making it appear pale and sallow.

Wrinkling and sagging on the surface of the skin actually reflect changes in the structures beneath it, primarily in the dermis. Here collagen tissues, which give the skin the strength to resist tearing when stretched, and elastin tissues, which allow the skin to spring back after stretching, become weakened. In addition, the skin itself and the fat layer beneath it both become thinner, and the dermo-epidermal junction flattens out—looking more like a serene lake than undulating ocean waves—adding to skin's fragility. These changes can make the skin look dull and listless on the surface. Thinner skin is also more prone to gravity and skin sagging, which can add to a droopier appearance.

It is possible to keep your skin looking younger longer by adopting good lifestyle habits. Don't smoke; drink alcohol only in moderation or not at all; avoid excess sun exposure; exercise and eat a well-balanced diet. In addition, use a moisturizer in your later years, which not only will help to counter dryness (another problem of aging skin) but will also plump up the skin, giving it, at least temporarily, a springier, more youthful appearance. There is also some evidence that estrogen replacement therapy may help to reduce the signs of aging in skin. One study found that estrogen increases the thickness in the epidermis of women who take it, but only for up to six months; after that time the improvement levels off. (For more medical research on treating aging skin, see Chapter 5.)

Some people just naturally age better than others do. Here's where those good family genes come in handy. People who have high cheekbones generally don't wrinkle or sag as profoundly as those who have rounder faces; because the skin has to stretch over the bone, there is less likelihood of wrinkling in the surrounding areas. In general, black women show the signs of aging less dramatically than Caucasian women, a difference that is thought to result, in part, from the greater amount of pigment in their skin, which offers protection against UV rays. Some studies indicate that black skin may have other natural antiaging properties that fairer skins do not have. For example, one study found that black skin contains more fibroblasts than Caucasian skin; fibroblasts are the cells in the dermal layer of the skin responsible for producing collagen and elastin, the supporting tissues of the skin. The collagen in black skin also appears to be arranged in tighter "bundles" than it is in Caucasian skin, which may offer more support to the skin.

Wrinkling is not the only skin problem that older women face. In addition to the fact that skin cancer lesions become more likely (see Chapter 2), there are other skin lesions that may develop as we age. Age spots, also known as liver spots, are flat, brown marks that may appear on the face, hands, back, and feet and are caused by sun exposure in older skin. Medically known as solar lentigines, they are harmless but may be cosmetically unappealing. Although there are over-the-counter "fade" creams available for these marks, they generally don't work very well. Sometimes dermatologists can remove lentigines by freezing them with liquid nitrogen or by applying a tiny amount of acid to peel away the lesion.

Many women also develop seborrheic keratoses with age.

These are brown or black raised growths that sometimes look like warts on the skin surface. Although they are not, in themselves, dangerous, they should be watched carefully; any changes or enlargement of these lesions may indicate that they are not seborrheic keratoses but early skin cancers that should be removed. Both you and your dermatologist should monitor these lesions carefully.

Cherry angiomas are small bright red or purple lesions caused by dilated blood vessels. They occur in 85 percent of middle-aged and elderly people, most commonly on the chest and back. Although they are not a medical concern, they can easily be removed in an office visit to a dermatologist.

While it's inevitable that your skin will show some signs of aging—as will the rest of you—more and more evidence has shown that your skin reflects your lifestyle. Take good care of yourself in general, and your skin will also look good right up to a ripe old age. And the fact that you'll also feel better inside will be reflected in a happier, more glowing face to show the world on the outside.

CHAPTER 2

Skin Cancer: Questions and Answers

Each year approximately 600,000 new cases of skin cancer are diagnosed in the United States, according to the Skin Cancer Foundation. In most cases the prognosis is encouraging; when detected and treated in an early stage, all forms of skin cancer have a cure rate of more than 90 percent.

But when skin cancer is left unattended, cure rates plummet, and the prognosis—particularly for the most serious type, malignant melanoma—can be disfigurement or even death. The news, alas, gets worse: skin cancer of all types is occurring in younger and younger people. Malignant melanoma is the leading cancer in Caucasian women between ages twenty-five and twenty-nine, and some research shows that women under age forty have a higher rate of malignant melanomas than men the same age. Afro-Americans have about 1/30 the rate of skin cancer that Caucasians have, but they, too, need to protect their skin.

Perhaps most tragic of all is the fact that most skin cancers are preventable if people simply avoid excess sun exposure. While in rare cases skin cancers can be caused by environmental hazards such as X-rays or exposure to certain chemicals such as arsenic, some doctors estimate that more than 95 percent of skin cancers are directly related to sun exposure.

The Three Faces of Skin Cancer

There are three forms of skin cancer. Basal cell cancer is the most common and least serious form. Squamous cell cancer is much less common but more serious. The numbers vary slightly depending on the person's race. Basal cell cancer is about five times more common in Caucasians than squamous cell cancer. But Afro-Americans are about equally as likely to get squamous cell cancer as they are to get basal cell cancer. Malignant melanoma is the least common (although, like all skin cancer, it is on the rise) but the most deadly form of skin cancer. Let's take a look at each of these types of skin cancer individually.

Basal Cell Cancer

Basal cell cancer (or carcinoma) affects one in eight Americans. Some of them are among our nation's most notable people, including Ronald Reagan and George and Barbara Bush. Although basal cell cancer used to be seen most often in older men (particularly those who worked outdoors most of their lives), the average age of onset of the disease has steadily decreased, and women now get it about as often as men. Ninety-five percent of all basal cell cancers are caused by chronic overexposure to sunlight. They occur most commonly on the face, ears, neck, scalp, shoulders and back (especially in men), and legs (especially in women), which are the areas most likely to receive sun exposure.

The basal cell layer of skin, where the cancer occurs, is the deepest layer of the epidermis (the top layer of skin). On the skin surface, basal cell cancer usually appears with one or more of the following five characteristics:

1. An open sore that bleeds, oozes, or crusts and remains open for three or more weeks.

2. A reddish patch or irritated area that may itch or hurt or cause no discomfort at all.
3. A smooth growth with an elevated, rolled border and an indentation in the center. As the growth slowly enlarges, tiny blood vessels may develop on the surface.
4. A shiny bump or nodule that is pearly or translucent and may range in color from pink, red, or white to tan, black, or brown.
5. A scarlike area—white, yellow, or waxy—which often has poorly defined borders. The skin itself may appear shiny and taut.

If detected and treated early, basal cell cancer has a 95 percent cure rate. Unlike squamous cell cancer and melanoma, it does not usually spread to other organs through the bloodstream, and it tends to grow fairly slowly.

Squamous Cell Cancer

Squamous cell cancer affects from 80,000 to 100,000 people each year, men more than twice as often as women. About 2 percent of the people who get squamous cell cancer will die from the disease. The cancer occurs in the squamous layer of skin, just above the basal layer. Unlike basal cell cancer, squamous cell cancer can be deadly if the tumors spread to other body parts. Between 1,500 to 2,100 deaths result from squamous cell cancer each year. But, as with basal cell cancer, 95 percent of all squamous cell cancers can be cured if detected and treated early. Here are some of the signs of squamous cell cancer.

Precancerous Signs

Certain precancerous symptoms are often associated with the later development of squamous cell cancer, including the following:

1. Actinic (solar) keratoses—rough, scaly, slightly raised growths that range in color from brown to red and in

size up to one inch in diameter. They appear most commonly in older people.

2. Actinic cheilitis—dry, cracking, scaly lips that may appear pale to white. This condition is caused by sun damage, which is why the more protruding lower lip is often more affected than the upper lip.
3. Leukoplakia—white patches on the tongue or inside of the mouth.
4. Bowen's disease—red-brown, scaly patches that may resemble psoriasis or eczema.

Signs of Squamous Cell Cancer

Like basal cell cancer, squamous cell cancer usually appears on chronically exposed areas of skin, which may also appear wrinkled and lax. Often these areas are protruding spots on the body, such as the ear, nose, lower lip, and hands. The following are among the signs to look for:

1. A persistent, scaly red patch with irregular borders that may crust or bleed.
2. An elevated growth with a central depression that occasionally bleeds. A growth of this type may rapidly increase in size.
3. A wartlike growth that crusts and occasionally bleeds.
4. An open sore that bleeds and crusts and persists for weeks.

Malignant Melanoma

If you want to know why dermatologists have been on the platform in recent years warning people off sunbathing, it is because melanoma is the fastest growing of all types of cancer in America. In 1935 your chance of contracting malignant melanoma was 1 in 1,500. Today your chance is 1 in 105. More than 32,000 cases are diagnosed yearly in the United States. By the year 2000, experts predict, 1 in every 75 Americans will develop a melanoma in his or her lifetime.

Although repeated sun exposure throughout one's life is thought to contribute to the development of malignant melanoma, in recent years doctors have determined that it is the serious, blistering sunburns in one's youth that can really set one up for developing melanoma in later years. In fact, one painful sunburn as a child doubles your risks for melanoma as an adult. And your risks increase with every sunburn you endured. So, even if you have sworn off sunbathing in your adult years, you may still be at risk for melanoma because of the indiscretions of your youth. Doctors say that a history of intermittent sun exposure is also a factor in your likelihood of developing melanoma. People who work indoors and spend much of their leisure time outdoors without wearing sunscreen, and those who live in moderately sunny climates (such as Seattle) and vacation regularly in tropical climates are at increased risk of developing melanoma.

The good news is that, diagnosed and treated early, malignant melanoma is more than 90 percent curable. Having regular skin examinations by your physician and doing monthly self-exams (more on this later) will help you to get an early diagnosis and improve your chance of total recovery. Of particular significance are changes in existing moles or the appearance of molelike lesions that did not exist before. Here are some important signs to look for:

The ABCDs of Melanoma

A. Note whether or not the lesion is **A**symmetrical. In normal moles an imaginary line drawn down the middle of the lesion will produce two equal halves. In malignant melanoma the two halves will be uneven.
B. Check the lesion for **B**order irregularity. Normal moles have rounded, well-defined borders; melanoma moles are irregularly shaped with poorly defined borders.
C. Examine the **C**olor of the lesion. Normal moles tend to be a uniform brown shade. Melanoma lesions tend to have more than one color—subtle shades of tans and

browns, black, and sometimes red, pink, white, and blue.
D. Consider the **D**iameter of the lesion. Average normal moles are about the size of a pencil eraser. Melanoma moles tend to be much larger, more than 6 millimeters in diameter.

Recently some skin cancer experts have added two more warning signs to the list, which can be designated as *E* and *U:*

E. Be alert to changes in the **E**levation of a lesion. Increased thickness and a lesion that looks more raised than it once did can be signs of a malignancy.
U. **U**lceration and crusting of a lesion are signs of advanced stages of melanoma that requires immediate medical attention.

What's Your Risk of Skin Cancer?

Doctors today say that there is virtually no one who is risk-free from skin cancer. Even dark-skinned individuals, once thought to be completely protected, can develop skin cancer if their skin is damaged enough by the sun. To determine who is most at risk, doctors have developed a technique called skin phototyping. The ability of the skin to burn is measured in the first forty-five to sixty minutes of sun exposure after skin has had no sun exposure. The lower your skin-type number, the greater your risk of photodamage and development of skin cancer. To gauge your own skin cancer risk, complete the following statement: "After my first exposure to summer sun for forty-five to sixty minutes, my skin will always . . ."

• Burn and never tan (skin type 1).

• Burn easily but tan minimally (skin type 2).

- Burn moderately but tan gradually and uniformly a light brown color (skin type 3).

- Burn minimally and tan well a moderate brown (skin type 4).

- Rarely burn and tan darkly (skin type 5).

- Never burn; my skin is deeply pigmented (black) (skin type 6).

Women with fair hair and skin and blue or green eyes are likely to fall into the first two categories. Women with olive or darker skin, dark brown or black hair, and brown eyes are likely to fall into the latter categories. Women with skin type 1 or 2 have a high risk of photodamage. Those with skin type 3 or 4 have a moderate risk, and those with skin type 5 or 6 have low risk. Notice that there is no such category as "no risk." Everyone is at risk.

Normal vs. Abnormal Moles

In addition to having a certain skin type, having certain moles may predispose you to a higher risk of skin cancer, especially melanoma. These moles have the medical name *Dysplastic nevi* (a term that means "abnormal moles"). How can you tell a normal mole from a dysplastic nevi? Here are some signs to watch for:

Normal Moles . . .

- Are unlikely to be present at birth but may develop any-time during one's life.

- Occur in about 80 percent of the white population.

- Are usually fairly small, less than the size of a pencil eraser.

- Are usually round with a regular border.

- Are flat or slightly elevated.

- Have a uniform color ranging from pink to dark brown or black.

Dysplastic Nevi (Abnormal Moles) . . .

- Are not present at birth but may develop anytime during one's life.

- Are larger than a pencil eraser.

- Usually have more than one color.

- Have irregular and poorly defined borders.

- May look more like an ink blot splotch on the skin than a round, defined shape.

- May be more elevated or look slightly swollen.

People who have many dysplastic nevi and/or have a family history of the moles are said to have the "dysplastic nevus syndrome," a condition that puts them at increased risk for melanoma. In general, most doctors believe that the more of these characteristics that appear in a mole, the greater the chance that it will develop into melanoma. Most dysplastic nevi never turn into melanoma. But doctors believe that people who do have many of these moles should have a complete skin exam every three to six months, and do monthly skin self-exams. In some cases removal of the moles may be recommended.

How to Do a Skin Exam

In addition to knowing your skin type and your sun exposure history, it's vitally important to do a thorough and careful skin self-exam once a month, beginning at an early age, to detect any lesions early. (Mothers should also do a monthly exam of their children, and husbands and wives should examine each other.) To do a skin self-exam, you need a full-length mirror and a hand mirror, a bright light, and a hand-held hair dryer. The American Cancer Society

and the Skin Cancer Foundation offer the following guidelines for doing a complete monthly skin exam:

1. Stand completely disrobed before a full-length mirror.
2. Examine your forearms.
3. Examine the backs of your arms.
4. Examine the front of your body, head to toe.
5. Examine each side of your body.
6. Examine the backs of your legs and buttocks.
7. Use the hand mirror and full-length mirror to examine
   your back. (This is where having a partner examine you
   is helpful.)
8. Using your blow dryer to separate your hair, examine
   your scalp—front, sides, and back (preferably with the
   help of a partner).
9. Using the hand mirror, examine the interior of your legs
   and genitals.
10. Examine the palms of your hands and the soles of
    your feet.

In addition to looking for the ABCDs of melanoma, you are
looking, in general, for any changes in a mole or existing
skin lesion. Persistent marks that you haven't always had,
painful lesions, or anything that bleeds, seems crusty, or ul-
cerous deserves immediate attention from your dermatologist. Any lesion that doesn't heal within a reasonable amount
of time should be checked by your doctor. Remember, again,
that the goal is early detection and early treatment.

How Is Skin Cancer Treated?

The first step in skin cancer treatment is a biopsy. The doctor
removes a small piece of tissue from the lesion and examines
it under a microscope. If cancerous tumor cells are found,
surgery to remove the lesion—and any affected skin around
it—is usually recommended. The type of treatment approach
will depend on the type and size of lesion, where it is located, and whether or not the cancer has spread.

The following are the most common methods of treating skin cancers.

Simple Excision. After applying local anesthesia, the physician uses a scalpel to remove the entire growth and a "safety margin" of normal skin, then closes the incision with stitches. Simple excision can often be used in the early stages of any type of skin cancer.

Electrosurgery (also known as curettage and electrodesiccation). The physician uses a sharp, ring-shaped instrument called a curette to scrape the cancerous tissue away from the skin, which has been anesthetized. Then an electric needle is used to burn the scraped area and a margin of normal skin around it. The two-step procedure is repeated several times, with the instruments going progressively deeper into the skin, until no tumor remains.

Cryosurgery. The tumor is removed by freezing with liquid nitrogen. This is often the treatment of choice for patients who cannot tolerate anesthesia or who have bleeding disorders. The procedure may need to be repeated several times at the same visit to ensure total destruction of malignant cells.

Mohs Surgery. This procedure was developed to help the surgeon remove all of a tumor while minimizing damage to the surrounding skin. The surgeon removes very thin layers of the tumor at a time and examines each layer under a microscope. This two-step process is repeated until the skin is tumor-free. Mohs is often used on tumors that have recurred and on those that are in locations that are difficult to treat, such as the nose, ears, and around the eyes.

Radiation. X-ray beams are directed at the tumor several times a week over one to four weeks until the tumor is destroyed. Radiation therapy is ideal for certain elderly patients and for individuals whose overall health is poor.

Laser Surgery. A laser beam is used either to excise the tumor, in the same way a scalpel would be used, or to destroy it by vaporization, in a procedure similar to electrosurgery. As with any skin operation using laser, one big advantage is that the laser seals blood vessels as it cuts, minimizing blood loss.

For advanced stages of melanoma and squamous cell cancers, treatments become much more invasive and, alas, less effective. In addition to removing the primary tumor, the surgeon may have to remove lymph nodes or other tissues to which the cancer may have spread. Standard chemotherapy treatments don't seem to work very well in treating melanoma. Researchers around the country are experimenting with many different systemic therapies. Some doctors are using drugs, such as interleukin-2, which can stimulate the body's own immune system to fight off cancer cells. Other researchers are investigating the possibilities of using retinoid drugs for fighting skin cancer. And some physicians are looking into combined therapies. So far, none of these therapies have provided an answer to the tragedy of skin cancer. Some researchers around the country are working on developing a melanoma vaccine, but for practical purposes the vaccine is still many years away.

As researchers become ever more frustrated in their efforts to beat skin cancers in their late stages, one fact becomes clearer: the best defense against skin cancer is to prevent it, by avoiding excess sun exposure and by making sunscreen use an integral part of your daily skin care routine.

Sorting Out Sunscreens

A generation ago people didn't really talk about sunscreens. The best sunscreen was a hat or a shady tree. Now sunscreens line drugstore shelves and have become big business. Yet, even as women accept sunscreens as a basic part of living in the 1990s, confusion still abounds. People continue to think there are good and bad ways to get a tan; experts respond that there is no such thing as a good tan. Many women still believe that they need many different kinds of sunscreens with many different SPFs; experts say that everyone should use one with an SPF of 15 or higher.

And many women believe that all sunscreens protect against all of the sun's rays; experts respond, not true—the type of screening depends on the ingredients used.

Sunlight: UVA vs. UVB

The first step in understanding a sunscreen is to understand just what you are trying to screen out. The sunlight that has been shown to be damaging to the skin is ultraviolet (UV) light. There are three types of ultraviolet light: UVA (the longest wavelengths of UV light); UVB (shorter, more intense wavelengths), and UVC (the shortest UV rays, not considered hazardous currently because they are filtered by the ozone layer; as the ozone layer continues to thin, however, some experts predict that UVC light could become a greater hazard to our skin).

On a sunny day about 95 percent of the UV radiation penetrating to the earth is UVA, and only about 5 percent is UVB. The ratio changes slightly throughout the day as UVB intensity builds toward noon, when the sun is directly overhead and UVB's shorter rays can reach the earth's surface more easily. That's why sunbathing between 10 A.M. and 2 P.M. is more hazardous than sun exposure earlier or later in the day.

Even though UVB is less prevalent than UVA, it is much more potent and, consequently, damaging to the skin. UVB used to be called the burning rays of the sun. According to John H. Epstein, M.D., clinical professor of dermatology at the University of California in San Francisco, UVB rays can penetrate into the epidermal and dermal layers of the skin, injuring the DNA, RNA, and protein in cells and damaging the walls of blood vessels. It can also damage the connective tissue in skin. "Initially, this will of course lead to the swelling and redness that are familiar as a sunburn," says Dr. Epstein, "but with repeated damage, the UVB rays are the most efficient cancer-inducing rays as well."

In contrast, UVA rays penetrate more deeply into the epidermal and dermal layers of the skin, but the damage they do is not as great. UVA used to be called the tanning rays, and they are generally the rays that are used in tanning booths and salons. Contrary to popular belief, however, even pure UVA rays cannot produce a "safe tan." Exposure to UVA can worsen the damage caused by UVB, and even on its own, UVA can cause damage to connective tissue in the skin that can lead to premature wrinkling. And the fact that we are exposed to so much more UVA throughout the day makes UVA a primary concern.

Understanding SPFs

It's important to understand just what your sunscreen can and cannot do. Virtually all sunscreens in the United States today carry an SPF number ranging from 2 to as high as 50. What does that number mean? Let's say that on your first venture outside for the summer season, you would normally become burned in 15 minutes if you were not wearing any sunscreen. Wearing a sunscreen with an SPF of 4 would enable you to stay outside four times as long, or 60 minutes, before your skin would burn. Similarly, an SPF 10 would give you 150 minutes and an SPF 20 would give you 300 minutes, or 5 hours, of protection. (Of course, to maintain that SPF while swimming, perspiring, and toweling off, you should reapply your sunscreen more frequently.)

But there's a catch: an SPF number reflects a sunscreen's ability to protect only against UVB rays. There is no guarantee that your SPF 4 is going to protect you for an hour from UVA rays; in fact, it's likely that UVA would be able to penetrate into your skin with only an SPF 4. "Most sunscreens with an SPF of 15 or higher are going to protect against both UVA and UVB rays, just because they are going to have the right combination of ingredients to screen out both UVA and UVB," says Darrell Rigel, M.D., associate professor of dermatology at New York University Medical School.

Just what are those ingredients? The following is a small

glossary of active sunscreen ingredients and what each of them does:

PABA (para-aminobenzoic acid), with its esters (glyceryl, padimate A, padimate O), is probably the most effective ingredient for screening UVB; it does not screen UVA. About 7 percent of the population is sensitive to PABA; they will break out in a stinging rash shortly after using a product that contains it and going out in the sun. Usually washing off the product and avoiding it in the future solves the problem. In contrast, all the other sunscreen ingredients combined sensitize only about 1 percent of the general population.

Benzophenones (oxybenzone, methoxybenzone, and sulfisobenzone) provide excellent protection against UVA but only minimal protection against UVB.

Cinnamates screen UVB but not as well as PABA.

Anthranilates are moderately effective at screening UVA and UVB.

Parsol 1789 (known by its long chemical name, butyl methoxydibenzoylmethane) is the most effective agent at screening UVA but does not screen UVB.

Titanium dioxide and zinc oxide are true sunblocks. They screen out both UVA and UVB by acting as a physical block on the skin, preventing penetration of UV light into the skin layers. They can also help to prevent penetration of infra-red light, the "heat" rays of the sun, which some doctors believe may be more harmful to skin than was once believed.

To determine whether your sunscreen provides full protection against both UVA and UVB, look for the term *broad spectrum* on the label and check for the right mix of the ingredients listed above. Also look for an SPF of at least 15. Cosmetics such as moisturizers and foundations that claim to contain sunscreen often have very low SPFs—as low as 4 or 6. If your cosmetic label doesn't have the SPF printed clearly, assume that the SPF is low and don't depend on it for total sun protection. Many women still have the notion that they should start out with a higher SPF in the beginning of the sun season and gradually lower their SPF as their skin becomes tan. Again the message should be clear: there is no such thing as a safe tan, so nothing but a high SPF should do.

Maximizing Sun Protection

Don't wait until you're sitting at the beach in the hot sun to apply your sunscreen. By the time you get settled and put it on, you may already have gotten too much sun exposure, and you're more likely to apply it unevenly.

For optimal absorption and protection, apply your sunscreen fifteen to thirty minutes *before* you venture outdoors. Most people need only about 1 ounce (a shot-glass full) of sunscreen to cover their entire bodies, but even coverage is a must. If you're going to be perspiring heavily or swimming, choose a waterproof sunscreen. According to FDA guidelines, for a sunscreen to be labeled waterproof or very water-resistant, it must maintain its SPF during an 80-minute submersion in water. Water-resistant sunscreens, on the other hand, need to maintain their SPF for just 40 minutes under water.

This does not mean that you don't need to reapply your sunscreen after your swim. Most people should reapply after perspiring or swimming if only because they are likely to wipe off quite a bit of the sunscreen when they towel dry. How do you check the "waterproofability" of a sunscreen? If water beads up on your skin after a swim (much the way it beads up on a just-waxed car), your sunscreen is probably still working. But it won't hurt to apply a bit more.

Since most sunscreens will sting if they get in your eyes during a swim or heavy perspiration, some doctors recommend wearing a wide-brimmed hat and sunglasses throughout a day at the beach rather than applying sunscreen to your forehead and eyes. Another option: try using a lip sunblock with an SPF of at least 15 around your eyes; the waxy structure of the block will resist running off into your eyes.

Don't reserve your sunscreen just for a day at the beach.

Doctors claim that most of us get more sun damage going about our day-to-day activities in the course of a year than we do in a two-week tropical vacation. If you don't want to apply sunscreen everyday, get used to wearing a wide-brimmed hat. Do apply sunscreen if you plan to spend any extensive time outdoors—during an alfresco lunch, for example, or on the ski slopes or while taking a walk. Your skin will thank you for it later.

Why Drugs and Sun Don't Mix

If you are taking any medications regularly, check with your doctor before spending time outdoors. Certain prescription medications—such as diuretics, anti-inflammatory drugs, and some antibiotics, including tetracycline—can cause skin to become unusually sensitive to sunlight, leading potentially to an extremely bad sunburn and/or hyperpigmentation of the skin. Certain perfumes and even certain juices—such as celery juice and the juice of some limes—can cause similar photosensitive reactions in skin. Often these reactions can be treated with topical hydrocortisone cream to reduce inflammation. Anyone who is using retinoic acid on the skin should avoid the sun entirely because use of Retin-A can lead to serious sunburns.

Self-Tanning Products

Doctors emphasize that we should be rethinking the whole idea that a tan gives one a "healthy" appearance. As one doctor said, a tan is like a hangover for the skin; it is a sign that the skin has had too much sun exposure, not that it's healthy. Most Americans are getting smarter, and the days of deep, dark tans are probably behind us. Even fashion models now are opting for no tan or only the lightest tan. Mothers, too, are starting to protect their children's skin more effectively beginning at an early age, habits that are sure to make the next generation more reasonable about sun exposure. Just as cigarette smoking used to be considered glamorous and is now regarded largely as a dirty, risky habit, so, predict many experts, will deeply tanned skin eventually be seen as evidence that one doesn't take care of oneself.

However, until society acknowledges the healthy appeal of our natural skin colors, many women will still want to look tan. Safer ways to go about it include applying some of the new bronzing powders to skin (many of which look quite natural) or using self-tanning creams, which today are much better products that those of yesterday, which tended to turn the skin a yellow-orange color rather than bronze.

Real vs. Fake Tans

A real tan results when the skin's pigment cells, which are located in the epidermis, produce increased pigment (melanin) in order to protect the skin from sunlight. The darkest tan, however, gives the skin only an SPF of about 4, which means that even tan skin can burn.

In contrast, self-tanning creams don't interact with the skin's pigment cells at all. They affect only the very top layer of skin, the stratum corneum. Self-tanning products contain a compound called dihydroxyacetone (DHA), which binds with the amino acids in the stratum corneum to produce a brown color that looks like a tan. The tan lasts as long as that top layer of skin does, a few days to a week. When the skin is shed, the tan disappears.

How to Use Self-Tanners

The results may vary depending on the product you choose, how well you apply it, and the natural color of your skin. You can increase the odds that the tan you get will be attractive by following these steps:

1. First exfoliate your skin before you apply the self-tanning product. Use a facecloth or loofah, along with soap and water, to rub away dead skin cells.
2. Apply the self-tanner according to directions in a well-

lit mirrored area to ensure that you get complete coverage; self-tanners that are poorly applied may result in unnatural-looking streaks.

3. Wash your hands immediately after applying the product so that the brown color doesn't occur in blotches on your hands.

4. Leave the product on as long as suggested in the directions, being careful not to rub or smudge the skin you're trying to "tan."

5. Realize that this new "tan" does not provide protection from the sun. Some self-tanners do contain sunscreen, and if you are going to be sitting in the sun, you should select one of them. But once you wash off the product, you will still need to use a sunscreen, just as you would if you had no color at all.

CHAPTER 3

Acne: Not for Teenagers Only

Most of us still associate acne with the "raging hormone years" of adolescence. In some ways that association is well deserved; acne affects three out of four teenagers, arising in puberty as a result of changing hormone levels, and it often dissipates by one's twenties.

Today doctors realize that adult acne is much more common than was once thought. According to some estimates, 27 percent of women and 34 percent of men ages fifteen to forty-four have active acne. Men are slightly more likely to get acne than women; for every five women with acne, there are eight men with the disease.

Acne in adults is the same basic disease as in teenagers, but it may appear slightly different. Some doctors have observed that in women acne tends to be most common on the chin, lower cheeks, jaw, and neck, whereas it is often most prevalent on the foreheads in teenagers. Acne rarely begins on the back and the chest in teenagers, as it does sometimes in adults. Some doctors believe that acne in adults is more resistant to standard treatments than acne in teenagers, perhaps because adult acne is usually a continuation of teenage acne—having lasted through many years, it is inherently likely to be more treatment resistant.

How Does Acne Occur?

Acne occurs in the hair follicles in the skin, especially those on the face, back, and chest. Each hair follicle contains a follicular canal up through which a hair grows. At the skin surface the opening of the canal is called a pore. Attached to the follicular canal are sebaceous, or oil, glands. These glands produce sebum (oil), which travels up the follicular canal to the skin surface and is shed onto the skin surface via the pore opening.

In a normal hair follicle, cells that line the follicle surrounding the hair are shed constantly and replaced. These cells are normally thin and wispy and are carried imperceptibly by the oil in the canal up to the skin surface, where they are washed away.

In skin with acne, the cells lining the follicle are sticky and adhere to the follicular wall, eventually causing a blockage of the follicle. The oil produced by the sebaceous gland becomes trapped behind the blockage and builds up. Bacteria present naturally in the follicle, particularly a type of bacteria known as *P. acnes,* become more plentiful because there is more oil on which the bacteria can feed. Over several days, even weeks, this blockage becomes inflamed and grows, producing blemishes. So the three "ingredients" in producing acne are (1) increased oil production, which leads to (2) more numerous bacteria, which are (3) blocked in the follicle by sticky cells that clump together.

Acne tends to appear first in adolescence because during the teenage years the body increases its output of sex hormones. Male hormones known as androgens, which are present in both men and women, are among those that are increased. Androgens stimulate the sebaceous glands, causing them to enlarge and increase their production of oil. Androgen production is greater in men than in women, which is why acne is more common in males than in females.

Acne is also thought to run in families; if your parents had acne, you are likely to get it too, but not necessarily. Emotional stress is also thought to worsen acne, although doctors aren't sure exactly how. It is possible that stress causes the body to produce more androgens and consequently more oil. Specific foods, such as peanut butter and chocolate, once thought to contribute to acne, are no longer considered factors in acne development, although in rare cases some people's sensitivity to certain foods could result in acne lesions. If your skin breaks out after every time you consume a particular food, you may indeed be sensitive to it and should avoid that food in the future.

Putting pressure on the skin can result in "friction acne," also called acne mechanica. It is often seen in athletes who have to wear padded equipment; football players, for example, often develop acne on their torsos in the shape of their shoulder pads; golfers sometimes develop a line of acne on their backs and chests where the padded strap of a golf bag presses against the skin. Even such mindless habits as resting your chin in your palm or cradling the telephone in your neck can aggravate or bring about acne.

Sometimes a product applied to the skin to make it look better—such as a moisturizer or foundation makeup—can actually make it look worse by increasing the likelihood that pores will clog. This is known as acne cosmetica. People with acne should avoid these products altogether or look for products that claim to be noncomedogenic (unlikely to clog pores), or nonacnegenic (unlikely to cause or aggravate acne).

What Kinds of Blemishes Does Acne Cause?

The initial blockage in the follicular canal is known as a microcomedo. As its name suggests, this lesion is so small that you won't notice it on the skin surface; it may be weeks before an actual blemish appears on the skin. Eventually, as the blockage enlarges and swells, a slight bump may appear on the surface of the skin; this is a closed comedo, or whitehead. In some cases, the blockage may cause the pore opening to stretch slightly open; the result is an open comedo, or blackhead. Contrary to popular belief, the black color of this lesion is not caused by dirt (and there's no reason to over-scrub your face to try to remove it). The black color results when pigment cells in the follicle come into contact with the air.

When a whitehead or blackhead grows too large or is squeezed, the follicle underneath the skin may burst, leading to a more serious type of blemish known as a papule. It is at this point that the skin surface surrounding a pimple can appear reddened and swollen. Once the follicle has released its substances into the surrounding skin tissue, the body's immune system sends white blood cells into this tissue, and these cells form pus. Such pus-filled inflammations are known as pustules. In severe acne blocked oil glands burst into surrounding tissue, causing inflammation and large blemishes known as cysts. These blemishes can cause permanent scars on the skin if they are not cared for properly, so they should always be brought to a dermatologist's attention.

These, then, are the five most common blemishes in acne: whiteheads, blackheads, papules, pustules, and cysts. While the latter three lesions are more disfiguring and serious than the initial two types of lesions, all of them are treated with basically the same medications.

How Should You Care for Acne-Prone Skin?

People with acne-prone skin, in trying to keep their skin as clean as possible, often overdo it because they think that if a little bit of something is good, more should be better. Often the exact opposite is true. Mild washing is great; nightly facial masks, and strong exfoliants for the skin may only cause irritation and inflammation and stimulate the oil glands even more. Here are some basic tips on caring for acne-prone skin:

1. Wash twice daily with a mild soap, using your fingertips to apply it to the face. Pat skin dry. Do not rub or scrub your skin.
2. Once your skin is clean, apply an over-the-counter or prescription medication as recommended by your dermatologist.
3. Be alert to your habits; try to keep your fingers off of your face and avoid manipulating your skin during the day.
4. Since hair can carry natural oils to your skin, adding to the oil buildup, wash your hair frequently to prevent excessive oil buildup. Develop a fondness for off-the-face hairstyles. Avoid putting styling gels, pomades, and lotions into your hair because they may also clog pores. (There's even a condition known as pomade acne, which occurs along the hairline as a result of using heavy pomades to control a hairstyle.)
5. Never squeeze a blemish. Tempting though it might be, picking or squeezing blemishes may result in pushing the contents of the blemish farther down in the skin. This can make the lesion become more inflamed and possibly infected.
6. Choose your cosmetics carefully. Apply moisturizer only when skin is really dry. Opt for lightweight lotions rather than heavy creams. Some doctors believe that women overuse moisturizers; many women with acne-prone skin don't need a facial moisturizer until they reach their thirties or forties. Choose water-based (not oil-based) foundations and powder blushers rather than creams. Look for sunscreens that have a clear gel, alcohol, or lotion base rather than creams.
7. Wash off your makeup before exercising. The combination of excessive perspiration and makeup can cause even a noncomedogenic makeup to clog pores. Wash your face gently after exercising to remove excess perspiration.
8. Avoid too much sun exposure. Although a light tan may

make you look better by covering some of the redness associated with acne, a tan will not help your acne and may even make it worse. Some doctors believe that sun exposure "thickens" the skin, making pore-clogging more likely. If you're going to be in the sun, wear a sunscreen with an alcohol or gel base rather than a lotion or cream.

9. See a dermatologist for acne that doesn't seem to be helped by good hygiene and over-the-counter acne products.

Making the Most of Visits to the Dermatologist

Tracing the causes of acne can be likened to solving the plot of a mystery. You can help your doctor in his investigation by planning ahead.

1. Keep a small notebook for a month or so, noting when you get acne flare-ups and the events that coincide with them. Do they tend to arise at a certain point in your menstrual cycle? Do they tend to occur when you're experiencing undue stress? Has your skin broken out more since you've had a baby or started taking oral contraceptives? Has your skin broken out more since you started using a new facial product or increased your sun exposure?

2. Bring all of your usual facial products into the doctor's office with you, complete with their ingredient labels. Sometimes acnelike flare-ups are really an irritant or allergic reaction to a particular ingredient or product.

3. Make note of any other skin conditions as well. Have you noticed more body hair than usual in recent months? Does your skin itch more than it used to? Have you recently experienced a sunburn or other skin assault?

4. Make sure your skin is clear of makeup and mois-

turizers when you visit your dermatologist. This may sound like an obvious point, but many dermatologists comment on the number of women who go to their checkups wearing makeup, which can interfere with a proper skin examination.

5. Once your doctor has begun prescribing medication, keep track of any side effects you experience, as well as how effective the product seems to be.

Acne Treatments: Which Is Best for You?

The good news about acne is that today it is more treatable than ever before. Dermatologists now have a better understanding of the causes of acne and therefore can address the problem on all three levels. There are medications that control the stickiness of the cells, preventing the blockages from occurring; there are drugs that can correct an underlying androgen excess in women and thus minimize oil production; and there are antibiotics that can reduce the proliferation of bacteria in the follicle. Some drugs are taken internally; some are used on the top of the skin. All of them work for some people, and most of them have some side effects. Here is a rundown of what your doctor might suggest using.

Nonprescription Medications

Just look on your drugstore shelves and you'll see dozens of products for treating acne. They are all likely to have one or more of the following "active" ingredients:

Sulfur (in Clearasil Adult Care and Almay Trouble Spotter, for example) works by curbing oil production.

Resorcinol and salicylic acid both help to exfoliate the skin, removing dead, scaly skin cells. They are found in many skin "toners" (often in combination with rubbing alcohol) and also in some acne medications (such as Stridex, Clearasil Adult Care, and Oxy Night Watch).

Benzoyl peroxide, one of the most well-known acne ingredients, is available in concentrations of 5 and 10 percent. It works by causing an increased rate of skin sloughing, helping to prevent the pores from becoming blocked by dead, scaly skin. Some doctors believe that benzoyl peroxide also can help reduce bacteria in the follicle. It's found in such preparations as Oxy-5 and Oxy-10.

Prescription Medications

Antibiotics

Basically there are two types of antibiotics for treating acne: topical (applied to the skin) and systemic (taken orally). In most cases of mild to moderate acne, doctors will prescribe topical antibiotics first. The two most common topical antibiotics used in the United States for acne are erythromycin and clindamycin. They are available in solutions ranging from gels and alcohol-based lotions to soothing lotions for skin that is easily irritated.

When topical antibiotics don't work to clear the skin, doctors may prescribe oral antibiotics. For women the use of oral antibiotics can pose a problem: many women develop vaginitis or vaginal yeast infections because the antibiotic changes the normal bacterial environment of the vagina. If you have had yeast infections in the past, particularly after using antibiotics, discuss this with your physician. Sometimes just switching to another type of antibiotic will clear your acne without causing vaginitis. (Of course, if vaginitis does occur it can usually be cleared up easily with an over-the-counter medication; it is not considered a serious problem, although it can cause intense discomfort.) Occasionally antibiotics produce some gastrointestinal distress. A few oral antibiotics may also raise your risk of photosensitive reactions: your skin may become highly sensitive to sun exposure while you're taking them. Discuss this possibility with your physician.

The antibiotics prescribed most commonly for acne are tetracycline and erythromycin. Some doctors may also prescribe minocycline, doxycycline, and trimethoprim-sulfa. Very occasionally oral doses of clindamycin are also prescribed. Most antibiotics can safely be taken for long periods of time, although as they begin to work, the dosages may be reduced.

Recently researchers have noted that certain strains of bacteria can, in some cases, become resistant to antibiotics, leading potentially to relapses of acne. Further explorations into this problem will undoubtedly lead to more choices in antibiotics in the future.

Drugs Derived from Vitamin A

You've most likely heard of Retin-A. It's been touted as the first real wrinkle remover, the first medical antiaging cream, a "miracle" drug. (For more information, see pages 85–86.)

In fact, Retin-A's first—and for a long time only—proven purpose was to treat acne. Retin-A (known medically as tretinoin) works in part through exfoliation of the skin; it loosens those sticky cells in the follicle, preventing them from forming new blockages. (Some studies also suggest that Retin-A has a regenerative effect on the skin; see Chapter 5.) Over 85 percent of acne sufferers who use Retin-A see improvement in twelve weeks. But Retin-A can cause redness and inflammation of the skin, especially in the initial weeks of usage, and throughout use of Retin-A it is vitally important to avoid sun exposure. Retin-A increases the skin's sensitivity to the sun and may lead to severe sunburns in people who use the drug and don't use a sunscreen. Retin-A is usually applied once daily or two or three times a week, usually at bedtime. It is available in gel, liquid, or cream form (the latter being for people whose skin becomes inflamed and reddened easily from the drug).

The other vitamin A–related drug that is used for acne is

Accutane (medical name, isotretinoin). Most doctors feel that Accutane is the most effective drug available for treating severe, treatment-resistant cystic acne. Nobody knows exactly how the drug works, but scientists have observed that sebaceous glands actually shrink when a patient takes Accutane, so that oil production is lessened.

For women, however, Accutane has one serious drawback: when taken during pregnancy—even once—the drug can cause extremely serious deformities in the developing fetus. For that reason most doctors will not prescribe Accutane unless a woman is using a highly effective means of contraception. Generally it is safe to try to become pregnant as little as six weeks after discontinuing Accutane therapy; the drug does not appear to affect the eggs in the ovary. Also, there is no evidence of increased risks of birth defects if a man impregnates a woman while he is taking the drug. Accutane can also cause side effects such as dryness of the lips, nose, and eyes, and because it has been known to raise triglyceride and cholesterol levels, Accutane is not recommended for people who have high cholesterol or a family or personal history of abnormal lipid metabolism.

Accutane is usually given in doses of 40 to 80 milligrams a day for about five months. At first the acne might actually appear a little worse, but usually the skin will start to improve by about the third month of treatment. Often improvement continues after Accutane therapy is completed, and about 40 percent of patients never need any acne treatment again. Most patients need only mild topical treatment. Relapses of acne are unusual after stopping Accutane therapy; if acne does return, it usually does so within three years and typically is not as bad as it was originally.

Antiandrogens—And Why Birth Control Pills May Help or Worsen Acne

In many women acne is caused by the fact that their bodies produce an excess of androgens, male hormones that in women are produced by the adrenal gland and the ovaries.

In some cases of androgen excess, acne is only one symptom of the problem. Others may include one or more of the following: hair loss on the head, excess body hair (hirsutism), menstrual irregularities, infertility, and polycystic ovaries. If you experience any of these symptoms, you would be wise to discuss them with both your dermatologist and your gynecologist.

Excessive androgens can sometimes be detected through a blood test, and often, though not always, doctors can identify whether the problem is the result of excessive output from the adrenal gland or the ovaries. If the problem is traced to the ovaries, your doctor may recommend that you go on oral contraceptives, which can suppress ovarian production of androgens. The birth control pill can either worsen or improve acne depending on the particular formulation of the pill. Pills that are relatively high in progestins and low in estrogens may actually worsen acne. So your doctor is likely to put you on a pill that is formulated to be relatively low in progestins and higher in estrogen.

For women who cannot tolerate the side effects of birth control pills, there are drugs known as gonadotropin-releasing hormone agonists, which suppress hormonal output from the pituitary gland. These are the "new kids on the block," and not many doctors use them. They can cause dramatic side effects in some women, including menopausal symptoms, and generally are reserved for severe cases of acne in women who cannot take birth control pills.

If the adrenal gland appears to be the main culprit in the androgen excess, your doctor may choose to treat you with very low doses of one of the corticosteroids, drugs that suppress adrenal gland activity. The corticosteroids most commonly used in the United States are prednisone and dexamethasone.

Some doctors also choose to treat acne caused by androgen excess with a drug called spironolactone. It is used most commonly in patients with high blood pressure because it is a diuretic and antihypertensive medication. Spironolactone is thought to clear acne by blocking the androgen receptors in the skin, preventing increased output of oil. It can, however, cause menstrual irregularities in about 40 percent of women who take it; this side effect can usually be prevented if a woman takes oral contraceptives at the same time she takes spironolactone.

With the exception of Accutane, acne could likely recur once use of any of these medications is stopped.

The Emotional Side of Acne

Perhaps the most important aspect to acne is how it makes you feel. Some women are not bothered by severe acne; others feel that they cannot leave the house if they have one or two blemishes. Today more and more doctors are realizing that acne is not only a skin disease; it can have profound effects on a woman's self-image and even on the things she does in her life. In one survey 45 percent of acne patients said they experienced great difficulty relating to other people. Another study found that the unemployment rate among acne patients was almost twice that of people without acne.

Even if you have only mild acne, if it prevents you from doing the things you want to do, you should consider visiting a dermatologist. You may discover that even a small improvement in your skin condition can be a big boost to your psyche.

CHAPTER 4

Beating Common Skin Problems

All skin conditions—serious or benign—have one thing in common: once you have symptoms, you want to know what the problem is and how you can fix it. Acne is the most common skin problem, and skin cancer, particularly malignant melanoma, is usually the most serious. But there are countless other conditions that cause skin symptoms. Although it would be foolish to try to cover every skin problem in one chapter, what follows are descriptions of some of the most common skin conditions, some of the current therapies for treatment, and where you can find more information on the subject.

Rash Remarks: Inflammatory Skin Conditions

Psoriasis

A chronic skin disease that causes scaly lesions in the skin, psoriasis affects between three and four million Americans— men and women equally. Psoriasis results from an overproduction of skin cells in the top layers of the skin. Although there are several different forms of psoriasis, the most common is called plaque psoriasis.

Normal skin replaces itself every twenty-eight to thirty days as maturing cells move from the bottom to the top layers of skin. But in the skin of someone with plaque psoriasis, skin cells mature every three or four days. The excess skin cells that are produced build up on the skin surface and form elevated red, scaly lesions. (In African-Americans, the skin patches may appear dark brown rather than red.) These lesions may be covered by dead cells that are continually being cast off, giving the skin a white or silvery appearance.

Plaque psoriasis may be mild (affecting 10 percent or less of the body), moderate (affecting 10 to 30 percent of the body), or severe (affecting more than 30 percent of the body). The skin patches may occur anywhere on the body but appear most commonly on the scalp, elbow, trunk, and genitals. The lesions can cause intense itching, dryness, skin cracking, swelling, and even pain.

Psoriasis is a highly variable disease. While it usually arises between ages fifteen and fifty-five, it can appear at any time in one's life. Often the disease first occurs after the skin has been injured in some way. Some people also believe that stress can trigger or worsen psoriasis. The condition can go into spontaneous remissions that may last for years, or it may steadily improve or worsen over time. About one-third of psoriasis sufferers have a family history of the disease, but the condition can skip several generations before showing up, so patients may be unaware that anyone else in their family has ever had psoriasis. Psoriasis can also vary with the seasons. Most people find that their psoriasis worsens in cold weather and improves during warm weather; doctors speculate that this is because the sun's ultraviolet light has been shown to be helpful in clearing psoriasis symptoms. (Psoriasis patients are often among the few people whom dermatologists actually encourage to spend time in the sun.)

Currently there is no cure for psoriasis, but there are some very effective treatments. Psoriasis is one of the most hotly researched skin diseases at the moment. New treatments and clues to the underlying causes of psoriasis could be around the corner.

Treatment for mild to moderate psoriasis usually begins with topical medications such as simple moisturizers, creams that contain cortisone, anthralin, and coal tar preparations. These may be used alone or in combination with controlled exposure to ultraviolet light. Treatments for severe psoriasis tend to be riskier than the topical therapies, and those risks have to be carefully measured against the benefits of treatment. They include ultraviolet light used alone or in combination with photosensitizing drugs known as psoralens; methotrexate, an anticancer drug that is given by injection or orally; injections of steroids; and retinoid therapies (such as Tegison and Accutane). All of these drugs produce side effects, which can be serious in some cases.

Doctors also suggest preventive techniques such as regularly taking whirlpool baths; minimizing contact with such irritants as soap and chemicals; reducing stress, especially by exercising regularly; using a humidifier in the home and the office, and protecting yourself from skin infections and injuries.

Currently doctors are having success in studies of psoriasis treated with drugs that are derivatives of vitamin D. Some researchers are trying to identify the gene that causes psoriasis; once that gene is discovered, a cure may not be far behind.

For more information regarding psoriasis—including different forms of the disease, psoriasis and pregnancy, and treatment options—contact the National Psoriasis Foundation, 6443 SW Beaverton Hwy., Suite 210, Portland, OR 97221, (503) 297-1545.

Eczema

Eczema is the lay term for what doctors call dermatitis. Dermatitis, which literally means "inflammation (-itis) of the skin" (derma), is used to describe any number of conditions in which a rash develops that may produce itching, swelling, blistering, oozing, scabbing, thickening, peeling, and sometimes darkening of the skin. The two most common types of dermatitis are atopic dermatitis and contact dermatitis.

Atopic Dermatitis

A skin disease that usually begins in infancy (affecting about 10 percent of all infants), atopic dermatitis clears up by young adulthood in all but 3 percent of people. It is part of a family of atopic conditions that also includes hay fever, asthma, and hives. If you have a history of one of these conditions, or if someone in your family has had atopic dermatitis, you are at higher risk of having atopic dermatitis as well. People with dry, sensitive skin are also more prone to atopic dermatitis.

Although no one knows just what causes atopic dermatitis, the following things are known to trigger flare-ups of the condition in someone who has it: exposure to certain irritating chemicals; ingestion of certain foods, such as milk, eggs, wheat, soy, and peanuts (these food reactions affect children almost exclusively); exposure to house dust; reductions in ambient humidity; exposure to harsh soaps and water; and illnesses such as colds, fevers, flu, sore throats, and ear infections.

In babies atopic dermatitis occurs most commonly on the face, scalp, neck, and diaper area. In adults it tends to arise most often on the face and in the folds of the skin at the elbows and knees.

Although there is no cure for atopic dermatitis, doctors can prescribe creams containing cortisone or similar anti-inflammatory ingredients, and oral antihistamines to minimize symptoms. It is also important to avoid contact with known irritants and soaps. Switch to a mild soap substitute for cleansing. Keep skin well lubricated with liberal use of a moisturizer, and use a humidifier if the air where you live or work is very dry.

Contact Dermatitis

If your skin has ever reacted to poison ivy, you have experienced contact dermatitis, which is simply a rash that occurs on skin that has been exposed either to an irritating substance or an allergenic substance.

Most (about 80 percent) contact dermatitis reactions are irritant reactions. That is, the skin reacts directly to an irritating substance by producing an itchy red rash. Examples of this type of contact dermatitis include skin that breaks out because of constant exposure to soap and water (for example, in people who wash dishes or bartenders who are constantly dipping their hands in the sink) or to irritating ingredients such as the alcohol in skin toners or the acetones in nail polish removers.

Allergic contact dermatitis, which is what poison ivy produces in skin, is more than just a skin reaction; it is, in a sense, a whole body reaction. It occurs when your skin comes into contact with an allergenic substance and your body's immune system recognizes it as a foreign substance and sends in the troops to fight it. In this case the "troops" are increased numbers of white bloods cells or, in cases where hives erupt, histamine. The white blood cells or histamine is what produces the rash. The following are specifics on the most common forms of allergic contact dermatitis:

Allergies to nickel. Many women experience their first allergic contact dermatitis when they have their ears pierced. The combination of injuring the earlobe (contact dermatitis is more likely to occur in broken skin) and inserting a metal earring can produce an itchy, weepy, swollen red rash on the lobes. These symptoms almost always signal an allergy to nickel, a common ingredient in most costume jewelry and even in gold jewelry. The rash usually clears up on its own once the earrings are removed, but thereafter a woman must be cautious about the kinds of earrings she wears. Hypoallergenic stainless steel earrings do not contain nickel, and high-quality gold earrings (14K or higher) usually contain only small quantities of nickel, not enough to cause a reaction. If you have an allergy to nickel, you should be aware of the presence of the metal in other objects, too, such as belt buckles, clothing snaps, watchbands, and garter belts. Nickel is also present in coins, but most people do not handle coins long enough to get a reaction. Cashiers, bank tellers, and other people who work with money, however, may be more susceptible to breakouts from exposure to the nickel in coins simply because they handle coins all day long.

Allergies to poison ivy, oak, and sumac. About 85 percent of the general population will experience an allergic reaction after contact with poison ivy, oak, or sumac. (Reactions to poison ivy and oak are most common; many sumac plants are nonpoisonous.) The best defense is to recognize and avoid the plants. The old maxim "Leaflets three, let them be!" is good to remember. On poison ivy and oak plants, three leaflets arise from a node on the stem. Poison sumac leaves consist of seven to thirteen paired leaflets along a straight midrib. These plants contain an oil called urushiol that interacts with skin proteins to produce an intensely itchy, blistering red rash several hours or even a few days after contact. Usually washing skin thoroughly with soap and water within 30 minutes of contact with the plant can prevent the reaction from occurring. You should also wash anything that has come into contact with the plant that you're likely to touch again, including gardening tools and gloves, clothes, and even your dog or cat. Recently some creams have come on the market that claim to prevent poison ivy reactions by serving as a block between the skin and the urushiol oil emitted by the plant. Early studies show that these can work for many people, and they may be a worthwhile investment for women who are highly allergic to these plants.

Allergies to cosmetics and fragrances. While cosmetics and perfumes are among the most common irritants and skin allergens (the preservatives and fragrances in cosmetics are particularly likely to produce a dermatitis in susceptible women), they can also be among the most difficult to identify. Women apply an average of twelve products to their skin daily, and manufacturers may change the formulation of a product without announcing it. So a moisturizer that you've used for five years may suddenly cause a reaction because it contains a new ingredient that your skin finds irritating. If your skin breaks out immediately after you introduce a new product to your skin care regimen, chances are you are reacting to something in that product; stop using it, and if your rash clears up, don't use it again. If, on the other hand, your skin starts reacting to products that you have been using for some time, stop using all of them for a week or so, then gradually introduce each product back into your skin care ritual, waiting a day or two after each to see if a rash erupts. When it does, it is likely caused by the product you've reintroduced that day; if you stop using it, your rash will most likely not recur.

If your rash persists despite these efforts, or if you simply cannot identify the source of an irritation or an allergen yourself, it's time to see your dermatologist, bringing with you all of the products you have recently applied to your skin. Your dermatologist may be able to do a patch test to determine whether you are experiencing an allergic or irritant reaction to an ingredient in one of your products. A patch test is done by applying a tiny amount of a substance to the skin on your forearm or back and covering it with a bandage-like patch. The doctor then checks under the patch at regular intervals, such as 24 or 48 hours, to see if you have reacted to the substance. If the test is positive, you are found to be allergic or sensitive to that substance.

Some areas of the skin—on the face, eyelids, and genitals —are more sensitive than others and are therefore more vulnerable to developing contact dermatitis than others. Skin that is broken or excessively dry has lost some of its protective barrier and is also more prone to contact dermatitis. Keeping skin well lubricated with moisturizers and avoiding known irritants and allergens are the best ways to prevent contact dermatitis. For persistent or severe reactions, your doctor may prescribe anti-inflammatory medications such as cortisone-containing creams to bring symptoms under control.

As discussed in Chapter 2, certain substances can also produce an itchy red dermatitis in skin in the presence of sunlight. In cases of photoallergic reactions (such as those to the PABA in sunscreens or to certain fragrances), the rash can take weeks to go away. Photoirritant reactions (such as those to the psoralens that are present naturally in limes, figs, parsley, and celery) can result in blisters and brown spots in the skin that may take months to resolve. The classic scenario for a photoirritant reaction is the woman who takes a Caribbean vacation and, while squeezing a lime into her pool- or beach-side gin and tonic, gets lime peel oil on her skin, which in the presence of sunlight can produce a nasty blistering reaction in some people.

The best prevention is to wash skin thoroughly before heading outdoors or at least immediately upon noticing a reaction beginning and to avoid use of the substance in the future. If the reaction persists or is severe, see a dermatologist.

For more information about eczema, contact the Eczema Association for Science and Education, 1221 SW Yamhill, Suite 303, Portland, OR 97205, (503) 228-4430.

Common Skin Infections

Viral Infections—Herpes, Warts, and "Water Warts"

While you may think of viruses as bugs that give you a headache, turn your stomach, and make you call in sick, certain viruses are likely to cause symptoms only in your skin. Some of them, such as herpes and warts, may stay for long periods of time or even permanently in a latent phase in which you have no symptoms but still have the virus. Others, such as the tongue-twisting molluscum contagiosum, which produces lesions that some people call water warts, disappear if successfully treated the first time around, usually never to be seen again. All viral infections that produce lesions in the skin can be worrisome to a woman who has to face the world with them and so deserve to be discussed. Also, skin viruses are common: almost one-quarter of all sexually active men and women in the United States have evidence of infection with herpes virus and/or papilloma virus (the one that causes warts). The following are more details on these three common viral infections of the skin.

The Many Faces of Herpes

There are two different types of herpes viruses: herpes simplex, which causes genital herpes and cold sores on the lips, and herpes zoster (sometimes called varicella zoster), which causes chicken pox and shingles. Both types of herpes viruses are spread by person-to-person contact. Herpes simplex is especially likely to be spread by intimate sexual contact; herpes zoster can be spread just by being in the same room with someone (as is evident by how fast a chicken pox epidemic can break out in an elementary school).

Herpes Simplex

Herpes simplex is caused by two very closely related viruses. They appear identical both on the skin surface and under a microscope, but scientists can distinguish them by the different proteins on their surfaces. Herpes simplex type I occurs most frequently on the mouth and lips; herpes simplex type II occurs most commonly in the genital and perianal area. (Note: Herpes cold sores on the lip are not related to canker sores that occur in the mouth; canker sores affect just about everyone at one time or another and are not caused by the herpes virus.) In fact, about 80 percent of genital herpes is herpes simplex type II, and only about 20 percent is herpes simplex type I. But it's important to realize that both forms of the virus can appear virtually anywhere on the skin, and it is possible to transmit the herpes virus from one's lip to one's genitals (through oral sex, for example, or by touching one's lips and then one's genitals) or to get herpes simplex type II on the lips by the same means.

For the most part, it's not important to know whether you have contracted herpes simplex I or II, except for the fact that if you have herpes simplex I in the genital area, you are less likely to experience frequent recurrences of the disease than if you have herpes simplex II; that can be of comfort to some women. If your doctor is affiliated with a lab where the technicians are skilled at growing herpes cultures, you may be able to have a biopsy of a lesion sent to the lab to find out the form of herpes simplex that you have contracted.

A herpes infection typically begins within one to two weeks of exposure to an infected person, but it can remain "hidden" in a latent state for months or even years. For this reason it can be difficult to pinpoint exactly who transferred the virus to whom. Women who have had more than one sexual partner over the years cannot assume that their current sexual partner gave them the disease.

Initial infections may be mild to the point of being symptom-free, or they may be severe. (Severe initial outbreaks of genital herpes are more likely in women than in men, although the reason is unknown.) The earliest symptom, which may appear about one day before the skin outbreak, is usually a feeling of itching or burning pain in the area where blisters will soon develop. In initial outbreaks this stinging sensation may be accompanied by slight fever, swelling of the lymph glands, headache, and muscle aches. The blisters will remain as blisters if left untouched, but in most cases they are broken through mechanical abrasion (moving the lips or, in the genital area, sexual intercourse, thighs rubbing together, or tight undergarments). The lesions appear as sores that will eventually crust over and dry up.

The most contagious period of the infection is from the time the itching, burning feeling first occurs until the crusts covering the sores have been lost (about seven days). Since many women have outbreaks that are completely asymptomatic (such as lesions that occur only on the cervix, where most women are unaware they exist), doctors recommend use of a condom during sexual intercourse to minimize the possibility of spread of the infection. In severe flare-ups of the virus, women may experience painful urination (with genital herpes), and the sores themselves can feel very painful for a few days.

Once a woman has recovered from an initial infection of herpes simplex, the virus goes into a latent phase in which it takes up residence in the nerve cells near the spinal cord. The virus may then stay inactive for months or even years but will never go away completely. The most common triggers for a recurrence of herpes simplex are trauma, depression of the immune response, and psychological stress. A "trauma" could be something as simple as sun exposure (on the lips) or intercourse or menstruation (for genital herpes). People who are immunosuppressed (such as women who have AIDS or cancer or who are taking systemic cortisone-like drugs) are also more susceptible to herpes recurrences. Periods of high stress in a person's life may also result in herpes flare-ups.

Prevention of recurrences, then, involves religious use of sunscreen (including lip balms with an SPF of 15 or higher) along with stress-reduction therapies such as exercise and relaxation techniques. Many women, particularly if they have severe recurrences, also take an antiviral drug known as acyclovir (brand name, Zovirax). This drug can be used either to lessen the severity of an outbreak (if it is taken at the very first symptoms) or to prevent future recurrences. The typical dose for prevention is three 200-milligram pills per day. Studies show that acyclovir can safely be taken for at least one year and possibly for as long as five years without any harm to the body. In fact, acyclovir is almost devoid of side effects when taken in this conventional dosage.

Herpes Zoster

Also called varicella zoster, herpes zoster is similar to herpes simplex in that once you have the virus, you always have it, although it will go into an inactive phase in your nerve cells. The vast majority of American men and women contract herpes zoster in the form of chicken pox during childhood, usually between ages five and eight. Less than 20 percent of the cases of chicken pox in the United States occur in adults.

Chicken pox lesions look like tiny fluid-filled blisters that usually first arise on the back, stomach, and chest but within hours or days generally spread all over the body, causing intense itching. Cases tend to be least severe in young children and most severe in adults, who may have, in addition to the blisters, severe headache, muscle aches, and a longer recuperation period. The disease is spread from physical contact with someone who has it or with something that the infected person has touched. There's also some evidence that the infection can be airborne, so that just spending time in the same room with someone with chicken pox could increase your risk of getting the disease.

The condition is most contagious from about one day before the blisters appear until the blisters have been crusted for about one week. Once you have been exposed to someone with chicken pox, an average of ten to twenty-one days will pass (a time span known as the incubation period) before you come down with the infection if, indeed, you do.

Treatment for chicken pox consists primarily of relieving the symptoms by applying a soothing lotion (such as calamine lotion) and taking oatmeal baths to minimize the itching. In adults and immunocompromised children, acyclovir is sometimes prescribed from the very first day of the outbreak; it can help to lessen the severity and the length of the disease when treatment is begun very early in the condition. Taking aspirin is strongly proscribed because the use of aspirin during chicken pox has been associated with the development of a serious condition known as Reye's syndrome.

Of more concern than chicken pox to many adults is the fact that once a woman has had chicken pox, she is at risk for developing a condition known as shingles later in life if the original varicella virus is somehow reactivated. More than

50 percent of people who get shingles are over age forty-five. The shingles rash is almost identical to that of chicken pox except that, instead of appearing all over the body (which occurs only rarely), it tends to follow the outline of the underlying affected nerve. In younger adults it occurs most commonly on the torso; in older adults it arises more often on the face and the scalp. The shingles rash can be intensely painful and can persist for two to three weeks, but especially in women over sixty, the pain may persist for months even after the rash has disappeared; this long-lasting pain is called postherpetic neuralgia.

Treatment for shingles consists primarily of taking acyclovir but in much higher doses than one would typically use for herpes simplex or for chicken pox. Some physicians may also prescribe steroid drugs to reduce inflammation. Taking soothing baths can help to minimize the itching.

Wart Worries

Warts are caused by a virus called the human papilloma virus, or HPV for short, and there are about sixty different types of HPV. The virus usually enters the skin through a tiny cut or abrasion. Some types of HPV flourish on the fingers, others on the feet, while others tend to take up residence in the genital area. Like herpes, HPV, once contracted, is believed to remain dormant in your body for years or even forever, possibly causing recurrent infections. But unlike herpes, which is believed to lie dormant in the nerve cells, HPV is believed to stay dormant in the skin cells in the mid portion of the epidermis.

HPV is spread by person-to-person contact or by touching an infected part of the body to a noninfected part. (Genital warts are spread most commonly through sexual intercourse.) It is unknown whether or not HPV can be transmitted from an inanimate object.

Warts can look different depending on the type of HPV and the location. Those on the feet (including plantar warts) are usually flat and calloused; genital warts usually appear in clusters of raised bumps; warts on the fingers and hands are usually raised rough surfaces. While they can be disfiguring, warts normally don't produce pain or other symptoms, except when they occur around a fingernail (periungual warts) or on the bottom of a foot, where the pressure of walking can bring on pain. Certain types of genital warts have been linked to an increased risk of cervical cancer, so women who have been diagnosed with HPV in the genital area are usually advised to have frequent Pap smears (about every six months) to monitor changes in the cervical cells.

Most warts clear up spontaneously even if you don't treat them, but many women want to treat them to remove them more quickly. Since there are no really successful medications for treating the HPV virus itself, the therapy for warts centers around removing them. You can buy over-the-counter wart removers that usually contain lactic acid or salicylic acid, which gradually dissolves the wart. Your doctor may be more successful using a similar but stronger solution of acids that induces peeling of the warts and the skin around them.

Warts can also be removed through cryosurgery (freezing with liquid nitrogen), curettage (removal with a curet—a sharp metal instrument with a circular end), electrodesiccation (in which a needle carrying an electrical current is inserted into the wart), or, in very severe cases, laser.

Some doctors even claim success using psychoanalysis and hypnotherapy to treat warts. The theory is that such therapy helps a person to rev up the immune system to fight off the virus. Or the therapy could have a placebo effect: you believe it can help, so it does. Placebo effects are thought to be behind the legendary success of such folkloric cures as sacrificing toads to clear up a wart. (Incidentally, contrary to popular myth, touching a toad won't cause you to get a wart.)

You may prevent getting the wart virus by keeping your feet well cared for and covered, bringing your own sterilized manicure utensils to a nail salon, and using a condom during sexual intercourse.

A Case of the "Water Warts"

Although not really a wart at all, the lesions that occur as a result of the common virus molluscum contagiosum are sometimes called water warts because their fleshlike coloring makes them look like watery blisters. This virus affects about 2 percent of the total population, causing small skin-colored or white dome-shaped lumps that are somewhat smaller than a common pencil eraser and may have a small indentation in the top. Unlike herpes and HPV, this virus is unlikely to recur if you've beaten it once.

Molluscum contagiosum used to be a disease that affected mostly children; today, because most transmission occurs during sexual contact and the lesions arise most commonly in the genital area, it is seen primarily in adults. The virus is not considered a health hazard in any way, although individual lesions may become inflamed and irritating.

The treatment for molluscum contagiosum is basically the same as that for warts—the lesions can be frozen off, destroyed chemically, excised, or, in rare instances, removed with electrosurgery or laser. Although ultimately the virus can be completely removed from the body, treatment can take several months because the virus has a long incubation period; even as the doctor removes some of the lesions successfully, the virus can be affecting neighboring skin, and other lesions can arise shortly thereafter.

Since molluscum contagiosum is neither a serious disease nor a particularly persistent one, prevention of transmission through use of a condom during intercourse is recommended, but not emphasized as strongly as with herpes or HPV.

Fungal Infections

Most common fungal infections in the skin are caused by one family of fungi called dermatophytes. These organisms are responsible for such common problems as ringworm, athlete's foot, and "jock itch" (known by the medical term *tinea cruris*). Ringworm is thought to be spread by person-to-person contact, but it is unknown exactly how one comes in contact with the fungi responsible for jock itch and athlete's foot. Certain people seem to have a tendency to develop fungal infections; other people may come into contact with the same fungus but not develop skin infections. Even people who are prone to fungal infections may develop rashes in only one part of the body; women with athlete's foot may have the infection only on one foot, for example.

All three infections can be treated with nonprescription antifungal creams (such as Miconazole or Clotrimazole) as well as prescription creams and oral antifungal medications (such as griseofulvin or ketoconazole). Treatment generally should continue for one week to ten days after symptoms have disappeared to ensure complete clearing of the organisms from the skin. Infections that cause severe inflammation are sometimes also treated with hydrocortisone creams to reduce the swelling. The following are symptoms and prevention tips to be aware of.

Ringworm

Ringworm is so named because the most telltale symptoms include a red, itchy, stinging rash in the shape of a ring. Many years ago it was believed that the rash was caused by little worms that curled up under the skin; today doctors know that the real culprit is a fungus that, like all fungi, loves to grow in moist, warm, dark environments. In adults ringworm is seen most commonly on the chest, back, arms, and legs and occasionally on the face. In children the condition occurs most often on the scalp and requires oral medication for cure. Once a doctor has diagnosed your problem as ringworm, you may be able to use a nonprescription antifungal cream to clear up the problem.

Athlete's Foot

A fungal infection, athlete's foot affects primarily the skin beneath and between the toes. The skin looks inflamed and cracked and feels itchy and burning. In the most severe cases (and the most difficult to treat), the infection also affects the nails, making them yellowed and thickened. If you've had athlete's foot in the past, you can help prevent future recurrences by wearing absorbent socks made from 100 percent cotton or from synthetic materials designed specifically to wick away moisture from the skin. Change your shoes and socks when they become damp, giving shoes at least twenty-four hours between wearings to air out. Applying antifungal powder to your feet a few times a day will help to keep them cool and dry.

Jock Itch

Although often associated with men, jock itch occurs in women too, causing an itchy, burning red rash in the groin area. If you've been treated once for the problem, prevent it in the future by wearing loose-fitting clothes made of fabrics that "breathe" (such as cotton) and by changing your undergarments when they become wet. Pantyhose can contribute to the problem in women by trapping heat and perspiration close to the skin; if you suspect this is true in your case, switch to stockings or knee-high hosiery. Sprinkling antifungal powder or even ordinary talc on the area a couple of times a day will also help to keep the skin cool and dry and thus less likely to encourage fungal growth.

Tinea Versicolor

About 5 percent of all fungal infections in the skin are caused by pityrosporum, a different fungus from those in the dermatophyte family, which is present naturally in your skin. When there's an overgrowth of this fungus, it can result in a condition known as tinea versicolor or pityriasis versicolor. The condition is seen most commonly on the chest, back, face, neck, and arms, where it causes white (or sometimes pink or brown), scaly spots about the size of dimes and nickels. Unlike other fungal infections, this condition usually doesn't itch or burn, and since it is medically harmless, treatment is usually just for cosmetic improvement. The condition is seen most commonly in dark-skinned individuals or in Caucasian women who notice the white spots when their skin gets a little tan in the summer. The condition can be treated with the same topical antifungal agents used to treat the other fungal infections mentioned above. In addition, many doctors recommend the use of shampoos that contain selenium sulfide on skin affected by tinea versicolor. These shampoos have a desquamating effect on the skin, meaning that they make the skin shed its dead cells more effectively, which can speed up the removal of the fungus as well.

Bacterial Infections

Unlike fungal infections, which can often be treated with nonprescription medications, bacterial skin infections almost always require a visit to the doctor for diagnosis and prescription medication. There are two types of bacteria that cause most bacterial infections in the skin: streptococci ("strep") and staphylococci ("staph"). Sometimes both types of bacteria are involved in the same infection. The good news is that the antibiotics used to treat bacterial infections are highly effective at fighting both types of bacteria. The following lists some of the most common bacterial infections of the skin, how to recognize them, and what to do about them.

Impetigo

The most common of all bacterial skin infections, impetigo affects children primarily. This is probably because adult immune systems are more successful at fighting the bacteria and because it is highly contagious and can spread quickly among the children in a school or day care center. Impetigo is caused by staph or strep organisms or sometimes both. When strep is the cause, children should be monitored carefully because in rare cases the disease may lead to kidney inflammation weeks after the infection has been cleared.

Symptoms of impetigo include small round blisters that turn into scaly, crusty lesions. The lesions can occur anywhere on the body but are most frequently seen around the nose and mouth. The infection affects only the stratum corneum layer of the skin and is not considered serious in most cases. Still, because it can spread so easily, treatment with oral or topical antibiotics and careful cleansing are usually recommended. In most cases impetigo infections when treated will clear up within seven to ten days.

Folliculitis

Literally "inflammation of the hair follicles," folliculitis is what some women are referring to when they use the term *razor bumps*. In fact, shaving or any repeated trauma to an area of skin is one of the most common spurs of this condition. Many women are familiar with the symptoms of folliculitis, even if they don't know the name: many small red bumps (papules) or pus bumps (pustules) in the hair follicle openings, where the hair meets the skin. In women the problem arises most commonly in the bikini area, caused by the combination of shaving the coarse hair in this area, the chafing of undergarments on the skin, and the increased perspiration in this area. The problem is also common on the legs. In many cases just stopping the behavior that's causing the problem (for example, taking a break from shaving) may enable the folliculitis to resolve on its own. Persistent folliculitis should be treated, however. Doctors may prescribe topical corticosteroids for the inflammation and topical or oral antibiotics to clear up any associated infection.

One of the most modern causes of folliculitis is the use of public hot tubs, and some doctors even use the term *hot tub folliculitis* to describe the rashlike symptoms that can result after time spent soaking in a hot tub. (The term *hot tub dermatitis* is also used to describe a rash in the skin due to hot tub use.) The heat and moisture provide an excellent breeding ground for the bacteria, especially a particular type of bacteria known as pseudomonas, which often causes hot tub folliculitis. In these cases the folliculitis commonly occurs on the trunk or the legs or arms. Again, antibiotics usually clear up the problem quickly but may not be necessary. To prevent reinfection, make sure that the water in the hot tub looks clean—avoid water that looks murky, oily, or has a persistent foam along the edges of the tub—and that the hot tub establishment follows regulations for cleanliness.

Boils

Perhaps the Bible's Job was the most notorious boil sufferer, but these very tender, red, inflamed lesions still affect many women today. Boils (known medically as furuncles) are hair follicles that have become infected by bacteria, usually staphylococcus. The lesion results when the body's immune system sends in white blood cells to fight the bacteria; the white blood cells combine with the bacteria and dead skin cells to form thick white or yellow pus. The lesion may throb and grow larger and more painful over several days. Boils occur most commonly on the scalp, face, underarms, trunk, buttocks, and groin area. Severe boils may cause fever and overall malaise.

Unusually large boils or boils that occur in clusters under the skin are known as carbuncles (or abscesses). These are much rarer than boils and should always be treated by a physician.

Many boils will burst or in some cases disperse into the skin on their own. Usually once a boil has burst, the pain is greatly reduced and healing occurs fairly quickly. Some women try to hasten the bursting of the boil by applying hot compresses to the area. Squeezing the lesion is not recommended because it can make the condition worse or even lead to a potentially dangerous condition if the bacteria get into the bloodstream. In some cases a doctor will make a small incision in the center of the boil to allow the pus to drain away, but usually taking oral antibiotics to kill the bacteria causes the lesion to disappear over several days without any kind of surgery.

Cellulitis

Contrary to some beliefs, cellulitis has no relation to the rippling look to skin that some women call cellulite (which, in fact, is just a term to describe what ordinary fat looks like at the skin surface).

Cellulitis is a skin infection usually caused by streptococcus bacteria that often enter the skin through a small cut or wound. Enzymes produced by the bacteria break down the skin cells, leading to symptoms on the skin surface that include a red, tender, swollen area about the size of the palm of one's hand. The infection, which arises most commonly on the legs and face, may affect the dermis layer of the skin primarily but can affect all layers of the skin and even penetrate into the fat and muscle layers below if left untreated. It can also produce high fever, weakness, chills, pain, and swelling of the lymph nodes. Cellulitis is always considered a serious infection, but when it occurs on the face, it is especially important to get help immediately because in severe cases the infection can potentially spread to the brain. When caught early, cellulitis can often be treated just with oral antibiotics. Severe cases may require hospitalization and use of intravenous antibiotics.

Pigmentation Problems

As discussed in Chapter 1, the color of your skin is determined by the amount of pigment (melanin) it contains. Melanin is produced by pigment cells in the skin called melanocytes. Although we all have approximately the same number of pigment cells in our skin, the melanocytes in dark-skinned people tend to be larger and to produce more pigment more quickly than the melanocytes in Caucasian skin. Certain conditions can cause these pigment cells to produce too much pigment (a problem known as hyperpigmentation) or too little pigment (hypopigmentation). Here are some of the most common pigmentation problems and what you can do about them.

Vitiligo and Other Forms of Hypopigmentation

Vitiligo is a condition in which, for unknown reasons, certain areas of the skin become depigmented, leaving patches of milky-white skin. The depigmentation can occur anywhere on the body, but common sites are the face, neck, and hands. Whereas in other hypopigmentation conditions the pigment production is simply diminished, in vitiligo it is believed that the melanocyte itself is destroyed, so that the skin, once depigmented, will never repigment spontaneously. About 1 to 2 percent of the general population is affected by vitiligo. The problem is associated most often with dark-skinned individuals, simply because the light patches of skin are more obvious against a dark background. The entertainer Michael Jackson is probably the most well-known vitiligo sufferer. In fact, vitiligo can affect people of all races and seems to be slightly more prevalent in women than in men.

The course that vitiligo takes seems to vary with the person who has the condition. Some people develop one or two white patches of skin early in life and never have any further sign of the disease, or they go for many years without change, then suddenly more skin becomes depigmented. In other people the disease spreads rampantly from onset until about 80 to 90 percent of the skin is depigmented.

Although the exact cause of vitiligo is unknown, some research suggests that the condition may be related to a dysfunction in the immune system. There is also some evidence that vitiligo runs in families; about one-third of vitiligo patients have family members who also have had the disease. Some experts believe that the pigment cells themselves are abnormal in patients with vitiligo.

Treatment for vitiligo consists of efforts either to repigment the skin or, if the vitiligo is very extensive, to completely depigment the skin. Depigmentation is accomplished through use of a prescription medication called monobenzylether of hydroquinone, which is applied topically and can destroy the remaining melanocytes. Repigmentation can be done through use of prescription topical corticosteroid drugs or with PUVA therapy (psoralen drugs plus exposure to UVA). It is thought that these drugs work by stimulating the melanocytes in hair follicles and along the edges of the depigmented areas to multiply, divide, and repigment the depigmented patches of skin. Some doctors also treat vitiligo by surgically transplanting pigmented areas of skin to the depigmented areas.

For small areas of depigmentation, the use of camouflage cosmetics (such as Dermablend or Covermark) or the application of self-tanning lotions can make the skin color look more uniform, at least temporarily. For more information about vitiligo, write to the National Vitiligo Foundation, Inc., P.O. Box 6337, Tyler, Texas 75711, or call (903) 534-2925.

Loss of skin pigment that is unrelated to vitiligo can result from injury to the skin, from some skin disorders (such as eczema and psoriasis), and from cryotherapy treatments (in which skin lesions are frozen off using liquid nitrogen).

Hyperpigmentation

In women some of the most common hyperpigmentation problems occur during the use of birth control pills and during pregnancy. It is thought that the changing hormone levels at these times contribute to the skin changes, although no one knows for certain.

Melasma (also called chloasma and "the mask of pregnancy") is a type of hyperpigmentation that occurs on the face in more than half of all pregnant women and in about one-third of women who take oral contraceptives. It is more likely to occur in dark-skinned women and in women who spend time in the sun. The condition is characterized by patches of darkened skin on the face—sometimes on the cheeks, sometimes around the nose, lips, and chin or on the forehead. In some women melasma clears up spontaneously within a year after they give birth, but it can persist for many years in women who have taken the birth control pill. Sometimes melasma affects only the top (epidermal) layer of the skin. This type of melasma responds fairly well to treatment, which includes bleaching creams containing the drug hydroquinone to lighten the patches of skin slightly, retinoic acid, corticosteroids, and sunscreens. Melasma that affects the deeper dermal layer of skin rarely improves with treatment.

Pregnant women typically experience darkening of other areas of their skin as well. In fact, almost no woman emerges from pregnancy without having had some change in pigment in certain areas of her skin. For example, the areolas (the pink area of skin around the nipples) typically darken during pregnancy and may remain permanently darkened afterward. Genital skin also darkens during pregnancy. Moles and other areas that are already deeply pigmented may become even darker. And many women, particularly those with darker skin and hair, develop a linea negra—that is, a dark line that travels from just below the breasts down to the navel—during pregnancy. This usually lightens over the next year or so after delivery.

Although most women don't seek treatment, the skin changes during pregnancy can be disconcerting. Just knowing that they are normal changes and that they will likely resolve on their own can be of comfort to many pregnant women.

Hyperpigmentation can also result from injury to the skin, from conditions such as eczema and psoriasis, and from the use of acne treatments. These types of changes are more common in black skin than in Caucasian skin. Patches of darkened skin can also occur in response to sun exposure after certain substances have been applied to the skin (for more information, see Chapter 2, pages 37–39.)

These small patches of darkened skin can sometimes be faded by applying lemon juice to the skin surface or by using a cream containing hydroquinone. People who have developed hyperpigmentation after skin trauma or acne should be careful to handle their skin very gently—not to scrub overvigorously during cleansing and never to pick their blemishes. These habits can raise the risks of hyperpigmentation in women who are prone to it.

Freckles and Age Spots

Pigment can also be deposited in the skin unevenly in the form of "freckles" in your youth (particularly if you are fair-skinned) or in the form of age spots (known medically as lentigines) as you age. Lentigines are caused by repeated unprotected sun exposure; the sun damages the pigment cells, causing them to produce too much pigment in little blotches. These lesions—and any lesion that erupts on the skin—should be watched carefully for changes that may signal skin cancer (see Chapter 2). In addition, women who already have freckles or lentigines should be especially careful to protect their skin from further sun damage by wearing a high-SPF sunscreen whenever they go out in the sun.

Freckles and lentigines can usually be camouflaged with careful makeup application. But for women who want a permanent solution to their blotchy skin, doctors can sometimes perform a chemical peel or dermabrasion (see Chapter 5, pages 81–85.)

Blood Vessel Problems

Some skin problems are not really conditions of the skin at all but are dysfunctions of the blood vessels that lie just below the skin surface. Two of the most common are rosacea and telangiectases (known commonly as broken blood vessels).

Rosacea

If you're fair-skinned and tend to blush when you eat spicy foods or indulge in alcohol or hot beverages such as coffee and tea, you may very well have an early or minor case of rosacea, a skin condition that is characterized by varying degrees of facial redness due to the enlargement and dilation of tiny blood vessels beneath the skin surface. Rosacea affects about one in every 500 people. In some cases the blood vessels in the eyes also become dilated, causing them to look "bloodshot." In severe cases rosacea can also lead to the appearance of a bulbous nose, a condition known as rhinophyma. (The actor W. C. Fields is the most notorious example of this condition.)

Sometimes rosacea can also cause acnelike papules and pustules in the skin, and for this reason many doctors refer to the condition as acne rosacea. But more and more doctors today believe that rosacea is really a problem of the blood vessels below the skin and, as such, is a completely different condition from acne, which has its roots in the hair follicles of the skin. Women with rosacea rarely have the blackheads and whiteheads associated with acne, and many medications intended for use in acne would actually worsen or irritate skin with rosacea.

Rosacea may actually be regarded as a cosmetic asset in one's youth, causing the "natural blush" that so many women yearn for. But over the years some blood vessels may become permanently dilated, causing a more persistent redness for which many women seek medical treatment. Although no one knows the exact cause of rosacea, some physicians believe that sun exposure can increase the damage to blood vessels, making them more likely to become permanently dilated. Emotional stress, temperature extremes (moving from a cold ski slope to the heat of a roaring fireplace, for example), alcohol, and some foods (especially those that are fermented, smoked, or marinated) can also bring on flares of rosacea and may contribute to the overall condition. Avoiding these triggers of the condition is the first step in treatment. Women with rosacea should also avoid topical skin products that contain high levels of alcohol, propylene glycol, and benzoyl peroxide, which can also cause blood vessels to dilate.

Doctors may prescribe oral antibiotics to treat rosacea, although physicians don't know for certain why they work in some people. Some doctors also prescribe a topical antibiotic called metronidazole, which is a gel developed specifically for treating rosacea. Severe cases of pustular rosacea can often be improved by the acne drug Accutane, but only women who take serious precautions against becoming pregnant should use Accutane because it can cause severe birth defects in a developing fetus when taken during pregnancy. (For more on Accutane, see Chapter 3, pages 48–49.)

"Broken Blood Vessels"

Whether you call them spider veins or broken blood vessels or the medical term telangiectases, the cause is basically the same: a blood vessel under the skin becomes permanently dilated, leaving a purplish splotch that shows up on the skin surface, looking perhaps like a spider or, in more severe cases, a small road map. These blood vessels show up most often in the legs and on the face. No one knows exactly what causes telangiectases to appear, but there's some evidence that hormone surges can play a role in their development because they often occur during pregnancy and the use of birth control pills. Long hours of standing, trauma to the skin, and a family or personal history of telangiectases can also make a person more prone to develop them. Telangiectases tend to be most common in women ages thirty to fifty, but they can also affect older and younger women and even some men.

Although telangiectases are not usually a medical concern, doctors can remove them for cosmetic reasons by injecting a sclerosing solution (some contain simply salt water; others use anesthetics) that inflames the blood vessel, making it swell and seal shut, no longer visible through the skin surface. However, bruising and, in rare cases, infection can result from the use of these solutions, and in some cases other telangiectases arise to replace the ones that have been successfully treated.

Keloids

Fleshy lesions caused by overgrown scar tissue, keloids often occur after the skin has been injured or experienced severe acne or even after a woman has had her ears pierced. Although no one knows the exact cause of these growths, they seem to be much more common in black individuals and East Asians than in Caucasian women, and there is some evidence that they are most likely to develop when skin is injured during periods of hormonal surges in a woman's life, such as puberty and pregnancy. Some doctors even recommend that if a woman has had keloids in the past, she should avoid having her ears pierced during adolescence and during pregnancy.

Treatment for keloids includes surgically removing the lesion and applying a pressure bandage (although there is a risk that another keloid—possibly even larger than the original—can grow in). Some doctors also try to shrink keloids by injecting cortisonelike solutions into the lesions. Once a woman has had a keloid, she should always inform her doctor of her scarring history before having any surgery done; sometimes use of pressure bandages after surgery can prevent keloids from forming.

CHAPTER 5

Anti Aging: What Really Works?

Americans are forever searching for the fountain of youth. In recent years that search has drawn women to cosmetic counters and plastic surgeons' offices around the country. But while over-the-counter creams and lotions won't take years off your face, you probably don't need to go to the other extreme and have a face-lift. There are nonsurgical approaches to removing wrinkles and "age spots" that can successfully make you look younger without all the risks, pain, and expense associated with surgery. Here is a rundown of some of your options.

Chemical Peels for "New" Skin

When the skin has many precancerous lesions and is also wrinkled, many doctors recommend a chemical peel as the best treatment. To do a chemical peel, the dermatologist or plastic surgeon applies an acid to the face. The acid penetrates down as far as the dermis layer of the skin, destroying the upper layers on its way. By removing those upper layers, a chemical peel smoothes out the skin, eliminating some wrinkles, lentigines, and precancerous lesions. There is also some evidence that chemical peels help to regenerate collagen in the dermal layer of skin; collagen helps to support and strengthen the skin, making it more resilient. Chemical peels may also remove excess elastin tissue, which can contribute to skin sagging. All of these changes help to make the skin look younger and "fresher."

Chemical peels do carry some risks, however, which vary depending on the type of acid used, the type of skin you have, and to some extent on the skill of the person applying the acid. Not all doctors are experienced in applying chemical peels; you should make sure that your doctor does this procedure on a fairly regular basis. Also, never have a chemical peel done by someone who is not a doctor; some beauticians around the country claim to do "rejuvenating peels"; steer clear. Cosmeticians do not have the expertise in skin biology and function necessary to do a safe chemical peel. (In fact, at this writing, the Food and Drug Administration is investigating the use of chemical peels by nondoctors.)

There are basically three types of chemical peels: light, medium, and deep. The lightest peels are often combinations of many different substances that may include retinoic acid, glycolic acid, resorcinol, and/or trichloroacetic acid (TCA). Most light peels penetrate only the upper layers of skin, reducing the appearance of fine lines, improving acne, fading pigmented lesions such as lentigines, and removing precancerous lesions. Some physicians prefer to do a light chemical peel several times over a year rather than one medium peel; risks are lessened, and the results on the skin surface are comparable.

Medium peels often require a stronger concentration of TCA, and the acid penetrates down to the upper layers of the dermis. Not only can medium-strength peels improve shallow acne scars and lessen the appearance of deep lines, but there's some evidence that they can actually promote new growth of collagen fibers, the tissues that give skin its strength and support. The results are also longer-lasting; whereas the results from a light peel may last for only about five years, the skin improvements from a medium-strength peel last about eight years. However, because medium-strength peels do penetrate down into the dermis layer of skin, the risk of scarring is increased. For this reason anyone who has a history of hypertrophic or keloid scars is not a good candidate for a medium or deep chemical peel.

Deep peels are performed by using a stronger acid called phenol, which is usually reserved only for women who want to remove deep lines and whose skin is very sun-damaged. Phenol penetrates deeply into the dermis, destroying as much as half of its layers. This peel can make even the deepest wrinkles less noticeable, as well as remove pigmented lesions and some acne scars, but the costs for such changes are high. Phenol is extremely painful during application and for about twenty-four hours afterward; medium and light peels are painful only momentarily, and the pain generally goes away after the procedure is over. In addition, phenol can penetrate the bloodstream and may cause damage to the liver or kidneys or lead to irregular heartbeats and other effects on the heart. Therefore patients must have constant cardiac monitoring while undergoing a phenol peel. Phenol may also completely depigment a woman's skin, so that she would likely have to wear heavy makeup to look cosmetically acceptable. For these reasons phenol is rarely used on any women who have dark skin because the depigmentation would be more obvious in this group, and it should never be used on people with pre-existing heart, liver, or kidney conditions or on pregnant women.

Recovery from a deep phenol chemical peel also takes significantly longer than from a medium or light peel. All three types of peels cause skin to look scaly and sunburned (the severity of the burn increasing with the depth of the peel) after the procedure is done. Many doctors wrap the skin in bandages designed to hold cold fluid inside, which helps keep the skin cool, reducing swelling and pain. Skin must also be washed with the gentlest cleanser and soothed with a petroleum jelly type of moisturizer. The skin heals by producing new layers of skin over the next few weeks. Recovery from light peels can take as little as one week; medium peels usually require two to three weeks before the skin looks presentable; but deep peels can require six to eight weeks for the swelling and redness to diminish.

Even the long-term care of skin changes after a chemical peel. Skin is more sensitive to sun exposure now, so daily use of a high-SPF sunscreen is more crucial than ever before. For some time after the peel, skin may also be more prone to infection, and healing will be slower. For this reason a woman needs to be especially careful to avoid any injuries to her skin and to have any skin infections she may develop promptly attended to by her physician.

Dermabrasion

Chemical peels can get rid of many kinds of facial imperfections, but they cannot eliminate deep scars on the skin, which are often produced by acne. Removal of these types of scars—as well as fine lines on the face—oftens requires the use of dermabrasion. In this procedure a doctor uses an electrical instrument with a diamond stone or a wire brush to scrape the outermost layer of skin until the skin is at a level at which the scars will be less visible. Deep scars may require two or three dermabrasions to be eliminated or reduced to a satisfactory level. Unlike chemical peels, which are usually done without anesthesia (especially light and medium peels), dermabrasion is generally done with anesthesia. Sometimes dermabrasion is combined with a chemical peel, in which case it is called chemabrasion.

After a dermabrasion, skin feels tingling, burning, and aching, symptoms that can usually be controlled with pain medication. The skin then crusts over as it begins to heal. Swelling lasts for about one week, and redness may last for several weeks, and it will be at least one week, maybe two, before you'll be allowed to wear makeup. This may be a good time to take some vacation time from work; by the time you return, you may really look like you've spent some time at the beach! Of course, as with a chemical peel, skin is more prone to infection and sun damage after a dermabrasion, so wearing sunscreen and being careful not to apply any contaminated products to the skin are vital.

Retinoic Acid: Youth in a Tube?

"At Last! A Medical Treatment For Skin Aging." So read the headline in an editorial of the *Journal of the American Medical Association* back in January of 1988 when the news that retinoic acid could improve fine wrinkling of the skin hit the airwaves and newspapers. Since then, however, there has been some controversy over just what Retin-A (the brand name for retinoic acid) can and cannot do. As of this writing, Retin-A has been approved only as an acne medication, not as a treatment for aging skin.

Retin-A is a cream or gel that contains tretinoin, a derivative of vitamin A, and therefore it belongs to the family of drugs known as retinoids. These drugs have been heavily researched in recent years for their potential uses for skin problems, including acne, hair loss, and psoriasis. Some studies indicate that with regular use (daily or several times a week) over six months or more, Retin-A can reduce fine lines on the skin and some deeper wrinkling, lessen mottled pigmentations of the skin, stimulate blood flow to give skin a rosy complexion, and reduce the prevalence of pre-cancerous lesions known as actinic keratoses. It works, in part, by providing a slow peel to the skin, stripping off the sun-damaged layers of skin to reveal the pink, healthier layers below. (This exfoliating effect is also thought to be one way that Retin-A helps to improve skin with acne.) There is also some evidence that Retin-A can penetrate deep into the dermis layer of the skin and promote the regeneration of collagen tissue, thus helping to build strength and resiliency in the skin from the inside out.

In April 1992 a dermatologic advisory committee recommended to the Food and Drug Administration that another tretinoin-containing drug, Renova, be approved for treatment of sun-damaged skin, including skin that is hyperpigmented, rough, and has fine wrinkles. Renova contains tretinoin in the same strength (.05%) as one of the three strengths in which Retin-A is available. But unlike Retin-A, which was intended for use in acne patients and therefore has an alcohol base in both its cream and gel forms, Renova, if it receives full approval by the FDA, will be available in a very emollient cream that is more appropriate for use by patients with dry, sun-damaged skin.

All of these potential improvements, however, come with risk. Use of Retin-A can cause severe redness and skin irritation in some people, which can usually be minimized by reducing the dosage and frequency of use, thus allowing the skin to adapt to the drug more slowly. Retin-A users also are much more susceptible to severe sunburns than the average person. (Some studies indicate that photosensitivity may gradually decrease with time and use.) Daily use of a high-SPF sunscreen is a must while a person is using Retin-A.

Not all doctors have greeted Retin-A with equal levels of enthusiasm. Whereas some doctors believe it truly may be an answer to wrinkling and aging in the skin, critics say that skin may look less wrinkled when a woman uses Retin-A simply because the skin is slightly swollen, making fine lines less apparent. Also, some physicians note that to sustain the effects of Retin-A, the drug must be used indefinitely, and the safety of long-term usage has yet to be proved. Retin-A is not recommended for use by pregnant women; although it has never been shown to produce problems during pregnancy, other retinoids are known to produce serious birth defects in developing fetuses when used during pregnancy.

Alpha-Hydroxy Acids: Retin-A Alternative?

Occurring naturally in fruits, sugar cane, and milk, alpha-hydroxy acids (AHAs) may be the reason why women as far back as Cleopatra were convinced that taking baths in milk and wine or indulging in fruity facial masks was good for the skin. These acids (which include glycolic acid, pyruvic acid, and lactic acid) have been found to aid in the treatment of acne, actinic keratoses, warts, and extremely dry skin, and may also diminish fine wrinkles and even out mottled skin. Like Retin-A, AHAs are thought to work by having a peeling effect on the skin, but unlike Retin-A, AHAs appear to achieve these effects with minimal skin irritation and without increasing one's photosensitivity.

Again, not all doctors are convinced of their efficacy. Some critics say that the effects are really dependent on the concentration of the acids; the higher the concentration, the more effective the product will be—but also the more likely it will cause irritation. Recently some moisturizers that contain very small levels of AHAs have become available without prescription; there is no solid scientific evidence that these over-the-counter products have the same effects as prescription doses of AHAs.

Injections for a Younger You?

When all else fails, there is always a magic bullet, right? That's what we'd all like. When it comes to antiaging, many women look for that bullet in the form of an injection. There are three materials that are generally used to fill in facial lines, wrinkles, and scars: collagen, Fibrel, and fat. (Silicone formerly was used but was never approved for this purpose by the FDA, and now most doctors have stopped using it.) Here is some information about each of the three injectable antiaging materials.

Collagen. Known by the trade names Zyderm and Zyplast, collagen is derived from the hides of cows. It is similar to, but not exactly like, the collagen in human skin. Collagen was approved by the FDA for injection into the skin in 1981 and since then has become the most popular injectable in the United States. Zyderm collagen is injected into the upper layers of the dermis to correct small surface lines such as "crow's feet" around the eyes. Zyplast collagen is injected into the middle and lower layers of the dermis to correct deeper wrinkles. The injections contain a local anesthetic for minimizing the pain upon injection.

About 2 percent of the general population is allergic to collagen, so most doctors perform at least two patch tests of collagen before injection to minimize the risks of an allergic reaction. There is some anecdotal evidence that collagen injections may precipitate the development of certain autoimmune diseases in some people, but this link has never been firmly proven scientifically. Corrections by collagen injection generally last only about six months before the material is absorbed by the body; repeated injections are necessary in order to sustain a correction, and these can be expensive.

Fibrel. A gelatin matrix implant, Fibrel is composed of three substances: a powdered gelatin made from collagen derived from pigs; aminocoproic acid; and the patient's own blood plasma. To have Fibrel injected into your skin, a small amount of your blood must first be drawn; the blood is separated in a centrifuge and the plasma used in the injection. Fibrel is used to correct deep furrows in the skin and some scars. It is thought to work not only by filling in depressions in the skin but by promoting the growth of collagen in the skin, so that even after the injected substance is absorbed by the body, the collagen will remain, and the correction will be longer-lasting. In fact, some studies show that injections of Fibrel can last five years or longer.

Although Fibrel carries virtually no risk of allergic response, bruising, swelling, burning, and pain upon injection are common, and the first three symptoms may last for seven days or so after injection. Also, fewer doctors are familiar with the use of Fibrel than with the use of collagen, so it is not used as widely as collagen. As with all injectables, the potential benefits depend in part on the skill of the physician injecting the substance.

Fat. To have fat injections done, small amounts of your own body fat are suctioned from your buttocks or thighs (not enough to be noticeable in these areas), and the fat is then reinjected into the fat layer of facial skin. Fat can be used to make only large corrections in the skin, such as filling in hollowed cheeks, because the needle necessary for injection is rather large. One big advantage of fat injections is that they do not produce allergies; one big disadvantage is that they rarely last beyond six months. In addition, bruising and swelling at the injection site may last for several weeks.

By now it's probably obvious to you that there is no problem-free, risk-free remedy for wrinkles and aging skin. In fact, the more researchers strive to find a cure for aging, the more evidence there is that the best defense against aging of the skin is to prevent it. Since about 80 percent of all skin aging is caused by sun exposure, not by natural aging, prevention begins and ends with the one nonprescription product that is a true antiaging cream: sunscreen.

CHAPTER 6

Drugstore Survival Guide for Your Skin

There is one thing you need to know about cosmetics: they are, by definition, not drugs. Therefore there are limits to what a cosmetic can do and what a manufacturer can claim a cosmetic can do. Keeping this one fact in mind will help you to understand even the most cryptic cosmetic promotions and to stand your ground with the most persuasive cosmetic salesperson.

Cosmetics are defined in the Federal Food, Drug, and Cosmetic (FD&C) Act as "articles intended to be applied to the human body for cleansing, beautifying, promoting attractiveness, or altering the appearance without affecting the body's structure or functions. Included in this definition are products such as skin creams, lotions, perfumes, lipsticks, fingernail polishes, eye and facial make-up, shampoos, permanent waves, hair colors, toothpastes, and deodorants."

Drugs, on the other hand, are defined as products "intended to treat or prevent disease, or affect the structure or functions of the human body." There are some cosmetics that are also drugs. Among them are fluoride toothpastes, sunscreens, antiperspirants that are also deodorants, and antidandruff shampoos.

Drugs are much more strictly regulated than cosmetics, and because they require more extensive premarket testing for safety and efficacy, they are much more expensive to produce. For this reason you will hear some executives from the biggest cosmetic firms claiming something akin to "our products today can do much more than we're allowed to say they can do." They'll say that their products can speed up cell renewal or promote skin healing or similar claims. You, as a consumer, have to realize that even when cosmetic companies have done premarket testing, these tests are not submitted to the Food and Drug Administration for review, and so, in the eyes of the FDA, there is no proof that a cosmetic can have any effects on the function of the skin. If it did, it would have to be called a drug and would come under the same scrutiny that a drug undergoes. Remember this anytime a cosmetic salesperson tries to claim that a product can do anything beyond just improving your appearance.

Choosing and Using Moisturizer

By the year 1995, Americans will spend approximately $3.5 billion annually on skin care products. Many of these products will be moisturizers. More than half of all moisturizers are hand and body lotions, and most of the remainder are for use on the face.

What Is a Moisturizer?

About 90 percent of all moisturizers on the market today are oil-in-water emulsions. This means that the product's major ingredient is water and it also contains an oil or oil-like substance (such as mineral oil, lanolin, glycerin, petrolatum, or urea) and an emulsifier (such as lecithin or stearates), which is an ingredient that prevents the water and oil from separating. Most moisturizers also contain preservatives, commonly parabens, and fragrance.

A small percentage of moisturizers are not emulsions at all but are pure ointments (such as zinc oxide and petroleum jelly), or they are based on high-tech delivery systems (such as liposomes, microscopic spheres that deliver water and oil to the skin in a "time-released" fashion).

Do You Really Need a Moisturizer?

The answer, most likely, is yes. A good moisturizing lotion is basic to a well-stocked medicine cabinet. Most women experience dry skin from time to time, and some experience it daily. When the skin gets dry, not only does it feel uncomfortable, but it is more likely to crack, thereby breaking down its protective barrier; in the worst case scenario, dry skin can lead to a greater risk of skin infection.

Moisturizers work by forming an occlusive film on the top of the skin that prevents water from evaporating from the top skin layers. Some moisturizers also contain humectants, ingredients that can actually draw moisture to the skin. Hyaluronic acid is a humectant used often in moisturizers today. In a sense a moisturizer acts as an adjunct to what your skin does naturally with the oil produced by the sebaceous glands. When that oil production starts slowing up, or the ambient air becomes very dry and pulls moisture from your skin, your skin may feel itchy and uncomfortable and you may need a moisturizer.

Most women need a body moisturizer, but contrary to popular belief, many women—particularly many premenopausal women—do not need a facial moisturizer. Consider the facts: the average woman has 600 sebaceous glands per cubic centimeter on her face, but she has only 20 sebaceous glands in the same area on her arms and legs. That's why the legs and arms are the first to feel dry. Hands can become especially dry if they are frequently exposed to soaps, which can strip away the skin's natural oils. In contrast, using moisturizers on your face, particularly if your sebaceous glands are producing enough oil already and/or if you're acne prone, might lead to pore blockage and potentially aggravate acne.

You probably don't need separate moisturizers for each

part of your body, however. Individual creams for your neck, eyes, and face usually can be replaced by just one good facial moisturizer. (Some experts note, in fact, that heavy eye creams worn at night may make your eyes look puffy in the morning.) Special night creams are also unnecessary unless you just like to wear a greasier product at night than would be suitable for day. It's probably not a good idea to use a body lotion on your face, though. Facial lotions are often formulated to be unlikely to sensitize skin or cause clogged pores. Lotions intended for use on the legs and arms—which are not usually acne-prone areas—may not be as carefully tested for comedogenicity. Most facial lotions are probably safe for use on your body, but since they usually cost more, it makes sense to purchase a separate body lotion.

How Much Should a Moisturizer Cost?

Today you can spend as little as a dollar or two on a drugstore brand moisturizer or more than one hundred dollars on a product from a well-known cosmetic manufacturer that is sold only in fine department stores. Part of what you're paying for when you buy the higher-priced moisturizer has no relationship to how well the product works; the higher price reflects the cost of advertising and promotion for the product. Who do you think pays for those top models' exclusive contracts? Most generic or drugstore-brand moisturizers have less advertising dollars spent on them, and that reduced cost is passed down to you as consumer. In addition, the following factors can also jack up the price of your moisturizer.

High-tech or high-quality ingredients. There are expensive oils, and there are cheap oils. Mineral oil and lanolin are among the least expensive lubricants used in moisturizers today, and for many people they are very effective. But a high concentration of mineral oil may aggravate acne in some women, and many women are allergic to lanolin. For these women it may be worth a little extra money to buy a moisturizer that contains vegetable oils instead—such as avocado oil, jojoba oil, and peach kernel oil (although, you should realize that it's possible to develop an allergy to one of these ingredients too).

Some of the new moisturizers contain ingredients designed to mimic the components of the skin's natural moisture barrier, such as fatty acids, lipids, and cholesterol. Cholesterol mimickers include such ingredients as squalane and cholesteryl isostearate. Cerebrosides are lipids found naturally in the skin but made synthetically by some manufacturers for use in moisturizers. Cosmetic manufacturers claim that these materials can boost the skin's ability to retain moisture. But some doctors point out that just because something is present in skin naturally doesn't mean that applying a product containing the same ingredients to the top of the skin is going to improve skin health or appearance. Furthermore, there is no solid scientific evidence that ingredients such as placental extract or collagen applied topically in moisturizers can have the rejuvenating effects on skin that some manufacturers claim.

New delivery systems. By now you've probably heard of liposomes. These microscopic hollow spheres in moisturizers usually contain oil and water as well as other ingredients, which, some manufacturers claim, are delivered to the skin in a "time-released" fashion over several hours. In this way the skin retains moisture for a longer period of time.

Again, solid scientific evidence for this claim is scant. Some women find that liposomes make for a more elegant product that goes on smoothly without excess oil. Liposomes may turn out to have real medical benefits too; some medical researchers are investigating their potential use as drug delivery systems through the skin.

Other moisturizers come in "serum" forms—single-dose applications that don't require preservatives because they're used fresh each time. These could be helpful for women who have allergies to preservatives in cosmetics, but for most women they're probably not worth the extra cost.

Botanicals. Plant extracts and essential oils have replaced synthetic ingredients in some products. For example, aloe and seaweed are sometimes used as humectants (substances that draw moisture to skin), replacing synthetic humectants such as glycerin, sugars (or saccharides), and hyaluronic acid. Plant extracts and oils can be more expensive than their synthetic counterparts, and their benefits may be negligible, especially if they appear toward the end of an ingredient list; anything that appears toward the end of a long ingredient list is likely to be present only in tiny amounts, possibly too little to have any therapeutic benefits.

Fragrances. Many products contain fragrance, which can be made synthetically (usually the least expensive method) or, in some of the higher-priced products, with essential oils that may or may not be more costly. (Rose oil, for example, is very costly; oil from thyme or rosemary is not.) Some women may prefer to have a fragrance-free product to minimize their risks of skin reaction and to lessen the chance that their moisturizer scent will interfere with the aroma of their perfume.

Behind-the-scenes research. Products from established, big-name companies are more likely to have undergone rigorous testing for sensitization to skin than those from fly-by-night companies. For this reason it's sometimes worthwhile to pay a little more for a product from a well-known manufacturer. However, often the generic or drugstore brand of a product is just as effective as its more expensive counterpart.

Pretty packages. Fortunately, the trend lately has been toward simpler packaging in cosmetics, both to reduce the price of the product and to make the package easier to be recycled (which many companies now offer). If you plan to display your moisturizer on your bedroom dresser, you may feel it's worth the extra money for an elaborate package, but don't judge the quality of the product inside by its outer appearance.

What may be important to consider is the sterility of the package. In general, cream moisturizers that come in a jar in which you dip your hand for every use can be easy breeding grounds for bacteria. A better alternative is to choose moisturizers in resealable tubes or pump dispensers to minimize the possibility of contamination.

How to Translate Moisturizer Claims

Manufacturers today are skilled at wording their moisturizing claims in just such a way that they won't get in trouble with the FDA but they might confuse the consumer. Here are some common claims on moisturizer labels and what they *really* mean.

"**Penetrates deeply.**" Well, not *that* deeply. Moisturizers can penetrate only into the top layers of the skin, and in fact that is all they need to do to be effective. The epidermis layer, which is constantly shedding cells and is exposed to the elements, is the only area of the skin that loses moisture on a regular basis. The dermis layer of the skin maintains a pretty stable base of 70 percent water; it doesn't need to be moisturized.

"**Minimizes the effects of aging.**" This is true to an extent. Moisturizers plump up the skin, making fine lines and creases less noticeable than when skin is dry. This effect is only temporary, however, and once you wash your skin or the moisturizer is absorbed or rubbed off, those lines may show up again. No ordinary moisturizer is going to make deep wrinkles or sagging skin disappear.

"**Protects skin from the environment.**" This probably means that the product contains a sunscreen, which is important protection if you are going to be out in the sun. Many moisturizers that contain sunscreen, however, provide only an SPF of 4 or so, which is not adequate protection for a full day in the sun. Look for moisturizers that specify their SPF. You can probably get better protection by using a sunscreen instead of an "antiaging" cream that contains a sunscreen, and you'll probably spend a lot less money.

Less well proven are claims of other environmentally protective ingredients such as "free-radical scavengers" and antioxidants. While it is true that free radicals—which are metabolic by-products—may cause cell damage, there is no hard evidence that chemicals that are applied to the skin can alter that process in any way.

"Contains vitamin A derivatives." This is usually put on products to make them sound like they have the same antiaging effects as the prescription cream retinoic acid. In fact, there is no evidence that the small amounts of vitamin A used in nonprescription moisturizers can provide any of the peeling effects of Retin-A.

"Fragrance-free" or "unscented." If you want to get a product that is less likely to sensitize your skin, choose the fragrance-free product. This means the product contains no fragrance ingredient or combination of fragrance ingredients. "Unscented" products may contain a masking scent—a fragrance that is put in the product not to bestow a particular aroma but rather to mask some of the possibly unpleasant natural odors of the other ingredients.

"Hypoallergenic." This term means that the product has been tested and found to be safe for use on sensitive skin.

"Noncomedogenic/nonacnegenic." These products are probably safe for use on acne-prone skin. Noncomedogenic means the product is unlikely to cause clogged pores. Nonacnegenic means the product has been found unlikely to aggravate existing acne.

Getting the Most from a Moisturizer

Once you've sorted through the options and chosen a moisturizer, the following guidelines may help you to make the best use of it:

- Apply moisturizer to legs and arms immediately after you shower or bathe, while the skin is still damp. The moisturizer will trap the water onto your skin and prevent excess evaporation of water from your skin.

- Here's a way to determine if you need a facial moisturizer: Wait ten to fifteen minutes after you wash your face in the morning and night. It's normal to have a "tight" feeling in your skin immediately after washing and doesn't necessarily mean you need to moisturize. If that tight feeling is gone within fifteen minutes, don't apply moisturizer.

- When possible, choose noncomedogenic, nonacnegenic moisturizers for your face. These products have been scientifically tested and been found to be unlikely to clog pores.

- Realize that even noncomedogenic moisturizers can become comedogenic if you layer them with other products. For example, if you apply a moisturizer, then a sunscreen, then a foundation to your skin, the combination of products could add up to clogging of your pores. Instead, consider eliminating at least one of these items by using a moisturizer with a built-in sunscreen, or a light, noncomedogenic sunscreen lotion in place of a moisturizer, or a moisturizing foundation. Another option is using a tinted moisturizer rather than a foundation for sheer, natural coverage.

- Always start small, applying just a little bit of moisturizer to form a thin layer. Too much moisturizer can become esthetically unappealing and may stain your clothes.

- Do not apply moisturizer to just-shaved skin, particularly in the bikini area. The moisturizer, combined with the open follicles, might cause a red bumpy rash called folliculitis. Wait at least overnight before applying moisturizer to shaved skin.

- For maximum penetration of moisturizer into hands and feet, apply moisturizing cream at night, then cover these areas with cotton gloves and socks for sleeping.

- If your skin tends to be dry, apply moisturizer to your skin before boarding a plane. The humidity in a plane is very low, and the drier air can pull moisture from your skin, making it feel tight and uncomfortable. A moisturizer will help to prevent this feeling.

Making the Most of Your Makeup

Even if you don't wear makeup everyday (although many women do), chances are you like having some around for special occasions or to change your look from time to time or to cover blemishes as they arise. Here is a complete guide to choosing and using your makeup.

Foundations: Back to Base-ics

Today most foundations—and most makeups in general—undergo rigorous premarketing tests to ensure that they are safe and unlikely to aggravate or cause any skin conditions. Still, choosing the right foundation for your skin is important in terms of minimizing acne and making your skin look great. Some doctors even point out that foundations can protect the skin because most of them contain titanium dioxide, a natural sunblock. Some also contain talc to absorb excess oil, and moisturizers to soothe dry skin. Here are some dos and don'ts on choosing and using foundation:

- If your skin is acne-prone, look for oil-free, water-based foundations that claim to be noncomedogenic and/or nonacnegenic.

- If your skin is dry, look for creamy moisturizing bases.

- Don't assume that you have to apply a moisturizer under your foundation. Try going a day without it to see if your skin seems dry; if it doesn't, you probably don't need the moisturizer.

- Don't try to match the color of your foundation to your skin color by testing it on your wrist; this color could be a shade or two different from the color of your facial skin. Instead, apply the color along your jawline and try to look in a mirror in the brightest light possible, preferably natural sunlight. For a perfect match, the foundation should blend completely into your jawline, with no line of demarcation.

- If your skin is pink-toned, try a basic beige formula with just a hint of pink; if your skin is yellowish, nonpink beige foundations are probably your best bet. Dark-skinned women should look for cosmetic lines that offer a wide range of darker foundation colors to ensure a good match to their own skin; some major cosmetic manufacturers have recently added lines of foundations specifically to match the many different tones in African-American skin.

- For light coverage you can apply foundation with your fingertips. Many women prefer the more thorough coverage that a makeup sponge affords them. If you use a makeup sponge, be sure to change it daily to prevent bacteria from building up on the sponge and being transferred to your skin. (You can buy bags of makeup sponges very inexpensively at cosmetic supply stores, discount drugstores, and variety stores.)

- If you only want to cover blemishes and not use foundation on your entire face, that's fine. Just be sure to blend the foundation well, particularly along the telltale jawline.

- For an overall look of flawlessness to the skin, many makeup experts suggest applying foundation with a sponge, then "setting" the foundation by applying loose facial powder with a large makeup brush. The powder gives the makeup a matte finish, which makes facial flaws less noticeable. Another option is to choose a foundation that specifically claims to have a "powder" finish. These products usually contain talc, which gives a matte finish to the skin surface.

- Foundation can sometimes double as undereye concealer —and may even work better. (Some undereye concealers can be too heavy and, if you perspire, may crease up under your eyes.) If you want to go this route, look for a foundation just a shade lighter than the one that you use all over your face. Blend the concealer down to your upper cheekbones, not just around your eyes, which can cause a "reverse raccoon" effect.

• Keep foundation looking fresh throughout the day by applying a lightweight pressed powder to oily areas—such as the forehead, nose, and chin—as needed. The powder absorbs excess oil, making your skin look smoother and silkier.

• To give eyeshadow and lipstick more staying powder, apply foundation to your lips and eyelids and top with translucent face powder before applying lipstick or eyeshadow.

Ways to a Beautiful Blush

Blush can add instant life to your face and make you look "healthy," even when you're feeling tired. The secret, of course, is to get the most natural look. Here are some tips:

• If your skin is acne-prone, opt for gel or powder blushers rather than heavier creams.

• Match your blush with your skin and hair color. If your natural hair color is champagne blond or brown, try peach, spice, rose, or cinnamon blushers. If your hair is golden blond or red, test out blushers in the honey, peach, and toast shades. Women with very dark skin and hair often look best with a berry, plum, or wine-colored blush.

• If possible, test blush on your cheeks, not on your hands, for the best match.

• If you use gel or cream blushers, try applying them under your foundation for the most natural effect. Powder blushers should always be applied over foundation, then, if you want, topped with translucent powder.

The Eyes Have It

The skin of your eye area is the thinnest skin on your body, making it also the most sensitive. Products that may work just fine on your feet and hands may cause a reaction in the eye area, which is why choosing eye makeup carefully is important, particularly if you wear contact lenses; flaking eye makeup can get caught under a lens and, in the worst cases, scratch the cornea of the eye. Doctors recommend that contact-lens wearers choose eye makeup designed specifically for use with contact lenses (which is less likely to contain ingredients that can flake off into the eyes). They also suggest that you put in your contact lenses before you make up your eyes, to minimize the chance of getting the makeup caught below the lens. Here are some more general guidelines for choosing and using eye makeup.

Eyeshadows generally come in three finishes: iridescent, frosted (sometimes called pearlized), and matte. As with foundations, the best finish for most women is matte. It is basically a combination of talc and pigment and is the least likely of the three types of shadows to irritate eyes. It can also de-emphasize the sometimes crepey skin in the eye area. Iridescent shadows give off a metallic shine because they contain ground metallic particles, which can sometimes irritate the eye skin. Frosted shadows may contain mica, or fish scale derivatives, which can also irritate the eyes. Both frosted and iridescent shadows may also accentuate lines in the eye area rather than diminishing them.

Eyeliners are available in the forms of pencils, cakes with a brush, or automatic liners in a tube. Cake eyeliners are less likely than the others to irritate the eyes, but they are also the most difficult to apply. Pencils are the easiest to use, but women tend to pull at the delicate eye skin more when they use them than when they use automatic eyeliners. Regardless of which type of product you choose, doctors warn that eyeliner should be applied only to the edge of the outer lids of the eyes, not to the inner lid, as has been fashionable. Lining the inner (usually lower) eyelids can increase the risk of irritation and infection to the eyes.

Mascara can offer the most dramatic enhancement to the eyes by playing up the natural length of a woman's lashes and making them frame her eyes more prominently. Ordinary mascaras tend to be mixtures of water, waxes, and pigment that coat the lashes, making them appear darker and longer. Waterproof mascaras replace the water with solvents, usually petroleum distillate. These are harder to remove but also last longer than water-based mascaras. Lash-lengthening mascaras usually contain fibers that can break off and irritate the eyes. Thickening mascaras sometimes contain talc or starch, which can also be irritating if they get in the eyes.

Eyelash and eyebrow dyes provide a longer-lasting enhancement of the eyes. The advantage is color that you don't have to apply and remove everyday and won't smudge or smear when you swim, cry, or get caught in the rain. However, these dyes do carry some risks. Eyebrow dyes are the same as semi-permanent hair dyes and, as such, carry some risks of allergy and irritation to the skin. Eyelash tints are silver-based metallic dyes that can be extremely irritating to some women. They should both be used with great caution and applied only by a professional in a salon.

Lip Service

Lips are actually mucous membranes, which require moisture and which contain little or none of the skin's protective pigment, melanin. For this reason they are highly susceptible to damage from excess sun exposure and dryness. Lipsticks, then, not only can make lips look more attractive but can help to keep them healthy. By keeping lips moisturized and protected from the sun, lipsticks (especially products that contain sunblock) prevent cracking and chapping of the lips

—problems that can lead to increased risk of infections or reactivation of infections such as herpes cold sores (see Chapter 3).

Lipsticks have three main ingredients: a non-water-soluble base, color, and fragrance. The base (usually comprising oils such as castor oil and lanolin) prevents the lipstick from being washed away when a woman wets her lips with saliva. The oils are mixed with waxes (such as candelilla wax) to make the lipstick solid and easy to apply. Color, the most important ingredient from an esthetic point of view, comes from dyes and ingredients called lakes, which are combinations of water-soluble dyes and such substances as white aluminum oxide that enable those dyes to be insoluble in both oil and water. (This is necessary to get the variety and brightness of colors in lipsticks; many dyes that are FDA approved for use on the skin are not allowed to be used in lipsticks because they may be harmful if ingested. The final ingredient is fragrance, used either to mask unpleasant odors (for example, from castor oil) or to give the lipstick a certain appealing scent.

When you choose a lipstick, most makeup pros suggest going for matte finishes for wear during the day and using frosted or iridescent finishes if you want a more glamorous look at night. Lipstick provides some sun protection by acting as a physical block to prevent UV penetration. But for maximum protection, use a lipstick with SPF 15 or higher or apply lipstick over a lip balm that contains a sunscreen.

Is Your Makeup Past Its Prime?

Nothing lasts forever, and even with preservatives your cosmetics eventually will deteriorate. Using them may even become potentially hazardous if they become contaminated with bacteria. As a general rule, the more water a makeup contains, the more frequently you need to replace it. The reason? Bacteria spread more easily in liquids, and infection can result. Store your makeup in a cool, dry place; hot, steamy rooms (like most bathrooms) may cause cosmetic ingredients to break down prematurely. Similarly, a clear makeup bag is great for helping you find things, but don't store it in a sunny place; the sun will penetrate right through the clear plastic, damaging the products. If you keep your makeup in a sunny spot, opt for an opaque fabric-covered makeup bag. Here's a quick timetable for giving your makeup a makeover.

- Every three to six months, replace your mascara.

- Every eighteen months to two years, replace creamy products such as moisturizers, concealers, blushers, liquid foundations, and lipsticks. (Replace them earlier if they start to discolor, if ingredients begin to separate when they didn't before, or if the product develops a funny smell.)

- Every two years or so, replace powder makeups such as blushers and eyeshadows.

Coming Clean: Skin Cleansing and Makeup Removal

Most women today don't really wash their faces to remove dirt; more likely what we're trying to remove is surface oils, makeup, dead skin cells, and some mild debris. Although three out of four women cleanse their faces with soap, this may not always be the best choice.

Choosing a Cleanser

Regardless of the type of cleanser you choose, make sure that it is targeted toward your specific skin type—oily, acne-prone, dry, sensitive. If you are unsure which cleanser is best for you, consult your dermatologist. Here are some of the cleansing options you'll be able to choose among.

Soap

Traditional soap is a combination of a strong alkaline product (such as sodium hydroxide or potassium hydroxide) and a weak fatty acid (such as caproic acid or oleic acid). Today many soaps also contain moisturizing ingredients and fragrances. Most soaps are fine for women who have no skin problems. Some may be too harsh for women with eczema, dry skin, or even acne-prone skin. It is never a good idea to use a deodorant soap, meant for use on the body, to cleanse your face. The soap is likely to be highly alkaline and may contain fragrances that could irritate the more delicate skin on your face, especially if your skin is dry or very sensitive.

Cleansing Creams

"Like removes like" is the principle on which cleansing creams work. The oil in the creams removes the oil on your skin and in your cosmetics. For this reason, if you wear a lot of makeup, using a cleansing cream will probably clean your face more thoroughly than ordinary soap. However, cleansing creams should not be used by women with very oily or acne-prone skin because they can leave behind a greasy residue. To remove that residue, regardless of your skin type, you may have to use a toner.

Toners

Also called astringents and clarifying lotions, toners are liquids that may contain alcohol, salicylic acid, resorcinol, and other ingredients that can cleanse the oily residue left over from makeup and cleansing creams. They can have a drying effect on the skin and therefore shouldn't be used on very dry skin unless they're followed by a moisturizer.

Eye Makeup Removers

Usually oily preparations, eye makeup removers are especially effective at clearing away stubborn waterproof mascaras that won't dissolve easily with soap and water. Since the eye area is drier than other areas of the face, even acne-prone women can usually use these products without adverse effects. Use eye makeup remover before you wash your face because some leave behind an oily residue that may be unpleasant and can be particularly bothersome for contact-lens wearers.

Facial Scrubs

Meant for use on oily acne-prone skin, facial scrubs include powders that you combine with water, as well as ready-to-use soapy products. They often contain tiny grains, typically of pumice or polyethylene. They can exfoliate the top layer of skin, giving skin a rosy pink glow, and they may help to control oil. However, too frequent use of facial scrubs often results in skin irritation. They should be used only two or three times a week, even by women with the oiliest skin, and they should not be used by women with dry or sensitive skin. Facial scrubs should never be used in the eye area.

Masks

Most women love to use masks; a facial mask forces you to relax for a few minutes while it dries, and therefore it's an indulgence. Facial masks generally come in one of two categories: hydrating masks (which may be gelatins, collagens, or peelable synthetic polymer bases) for dry skin and oil-absorbing masks (usually in bases of clay or mud) for acne-prone or oily skin. In addition, they may contain fragrances and natural botanical ingredients to add to the esthetic experience of wearing one. Because they exfoliate the top layer of skin, masks can make the skin feel smoother and softer and may give a rosy glow to the skin by stimulating blood flow to the skin surface. These effects are temporary. Masks alone will not clear up acne, erase wrinkles, or remove body "toxins," as is sometimes claimed. Most masks should be left on the skin for no longer than five minutes or so, and they should be removed gently, with splashes of water and perhaps gentle rubbing with a facecloth. Rough removal of a mask will irritate the skin. Most masks should also not be applied more than once or twice a week.

Good, Basic Cleansing

If you have any chronic skin problems—such as acne, eczema, or psoriasis—it's best to consult your dermatologist about the best cleansing routine for you. Most women who heed the following tips should be able to cleanse their skin successfully and with minimal problems.

- Cleanse your skin twice a day—once in the morning, to remove oils that have accumulated at night and to prepare the skin for makeup, and once at night, to remove makeup and surface oils and debris.

- Never go to sleep with makeup on your face; not only will you smudge your pillowcases, but you may clog your pores.

- Remove makeup before engaging in strenuous exercise. The combination of perspiration and cosmetics can lead to clogged pores. If you can't wash before your workout, at least make sure to cleanse your skin immediately after you exercise to remove makeup, perspiration, and oils.

- When in doubt, do less than you think you need. Go with the more gentle soap, use your fingertips instead of a facecloth, never rub too hard. You are more likely to irritate your skin from overcleansing than to cleanse too little.

- If your skin is sensitive, look for fragrance-free soaps and cleansers, which are less likely to cause an irritation.

- Wash with lukewarm water. Water that is too hot or too cold can also irritate the skin.

- Rinse your skin thoroughly, splashing at least fifteen times with water. Cleanser residue can be unappealing and may irritate the skin.

- Remember to wash your neck too, especially if you have applied makeup down below your jawline.

PART II

Beautiful Hair

CHAPTER 7

The Five Ages of Hair

The look and feel of a woman's hair is tied into the very essence of what it is to be female. In fact, women, more than men, are often described simply by virtue of their hair: a "fiery redhead," a "dizzy blond," a "raven-haired beauty." While many of us cringe at being summed up in such superficial terms, the very fact that these descriptions are so familiar points up the integral part that hair plays in one's womanhood. Little wonder, then, that we become so dismayed over bad haircuts and hair coloring or perms that went wrong. When your hair looks bad, it is hard to feel good about your appearance. And if you don't feel good about the way you look, it may be hard to muster the confidence or energy needed to go about your day-to-day responsibilities with a sense of pride. The often-heard expression "Leave me alone—I'm having a bad hair day," while usually said in jest, may be a justifiable complaint for many women.

Good grooming begins at the top, with your hair, and there's no better place to start than with a basic understanding of what your hair is, how it is likely to change throughout your life, and what you can do to make it look its best.

The Anatomy of Hair

Hair is made of the same proteinous substance—keratin—that comprises the nails and the top, stratum corneum layer of the skin. While hair is composed of dead cells, its growth and reproduction are spurred by living cells at the base of the hair follicles, known as the hair root. The hair root is located deep in the dermis layer of the skin. The hair itself, or the hair "shaft," grows up through the follicle, which is lubricated by an adjoining sebaceous (oil) gland, through the dermis and epidermis to the surface of the skin, where it emerges through the follicle opening, known as the pore. The average person has about 100,000 hair follicles on the head, and each produces a single hair.

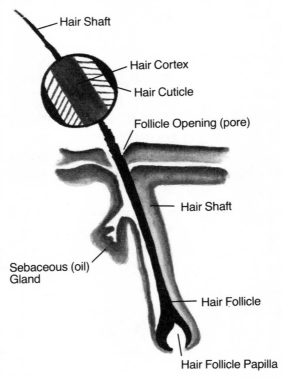

Hair Shaft

Hair Cortex

Hair Cuticle

Follicle Opening (pore)

Hair Shaft

Sebaceous (oil) Gland

Hair Follicle

Hair Follicle Papilla

As you probably know, humans, like all mammals, are covered with hair, virtually all over our bodies (except for the palms of our hands, soles of our feet, tips of our toes and fingers, and parts of our genitals). In women most of this hair is soft vellus hair that is barely perceptible in some areas (such as the "peach fuzz" on one's facial cheeks). The hair that is noticeable—on our heads, genitals, underarms, legs, arms, eyebrows and lashes, and sometimes on other body parts—is known as terminal hair. Unlike vellus hairs, which are soft and unpigmented, terminal hairs are coarser and stronger and contain pigment, which may vary slightly on different areas of the body. Throughout the rest of this section of the book, the hair we will be referring to will be the terminal hairs.

Hair, like skin, is composed of two primary layers. The cuticle layer is the outer layer. Just as the epidermis protects the dermis layer of the skin, the cuticle layer's main function is to protect the important inner layer of the hair, the cortex, which supports the hair shaft and also contains the hair pigment, melanin. There are two types of melanin: eumelanin is a brownish-black pigment that is present in all hair colors, blond through black, in varying amounts; pheomelanin is a red-yellow pigment that is thought also to be present in all hair colors but predominates in people with naturally red or blond hair. (Gray hair is really hair that has no pigment.)

The cuticle is composed of several tiny layers of overlapping cells, which are lined up, it is often said, like shingles on a roof or like scales on a fish. In healthy, "virgin" hair, the shingles lie flat, making the hair reflect light well and hence giving hair its shine. In hair that has been damaged—through use of heated styling tools; coloring, straightening, or perming chemicals; or even too-vigorous brushing and combing —this cuticle can become "roughened up," making the hair look duller and causing it to tangle more easily. Also, as when the skin barrier is broken through injury, the barrier layer of the hair has also been damaged, making the hair more porous and more susceptible to the negative effects of further chemical processes and heat.

Hair is forever regenerating itself (except hair that comes from follicles that ultimately stop producing—see Chapter 9, pages 142–145.) This means that the damage you cause your hair today may be overcome fairly easily by treating your hair carefully. Basic tips such as keeping hair clean, getting regular trims, not overstyling, avoiding repeated applications of coloring and perming chemicals to the same hair shafts, and taking care of hair problems when they first occur all can help you to keep your hair looking and feeling healthy throughout your life.

The Five Ages of Your Hair

Knowing what changes to expect in your hair as you age can also help. The following is a basic description of the life cycle of a head of hair.

Infancy

In a fetus the hair follicles and oil glands are formed by the sixth month, and there is most likely a fine growth of hair on the head and possibly over the back and shoulders. The color of this hair may or may not resemble the color the hair will be later in life. Most babies are born with a soft, downy head of hair that usually lasts only the first three months or so after birth. During this time the hair gradually falls out for unknown reasons, and new hair grows in, usually in a much fuller and uniform pattern. Interestingly, this pattern of hair loss and regrowth parallels a similar pattern in the new mother, who often notices increased shedding of her hair about three months after childbirth but by six months post-partum has usually returned to a normal growing and shedding schedule.

Since most children go through their first year of life with little hair, the care of this hair is relatively simple—shampooing when necessary and trimming to keep hair out of the eyes and to minimize tangling. Most pediatricians recommend using a baby shampoo during the first few years of a child's life. These shampoos don't contain the sulfates used in most adult shampoos, which can sting the eyes if they drift down from the scalp.

Some children in the very first few months of life may experience scaliness and redness of the scalp. This condition is known as cradle cap and is actually fairly common. When the redness and scaliness are also found on the face and/or the diaper area, it is known as seborrheic dermatitis (for more on seborrheic dermatitis in adults, see Chapter 9, page 148). In most infants cradle cap resolves within a few months without any treatment. It is not thought to produce itch or discomfort in infants. Cradle cap can usually be treated by washing the baby's hair with baby shampoo (perhaps slightly more frequently than usual) and brushing to loosen the scales. If the symptoms also occur on the face and/or diaper area (indicating seborrheic dermatitis), they should be reported to the pediatrician. The doctor may prescribe an ointment containing hydrocortisone to reduce inflammation for this condition and may also recommend use of a stronger, antiseborrheic shampoo.

Childhood

As a baby grows into a child, her hair, which may have been light blond when she was an infant and toddler, may start to turn darker. Although no one knows exactly why this happens, it is believed that the pigment cells gradually mature and produce more pigment over the early years of childhood, placing increased pigment not only in the hair of the child but even possibly in the skin. In fact, some black children are born with quite light-colored skin and hair but usually have fully pigmented hair and skin by the time they become toddlers.

Hairstyle preferences may also start to surface in childhood and continue throughout the teens. Many a parent can relate stories of arguments over whether or not their child would wear a ponytail to school or some other seemingly trivial matter. This is the age to begin to encourage your child to follow good hair hygiene, by "investing" in fun clips and elastic bands to keep your child's hair neat, off her face, and less likely to tangle. (Stay away from clips with sharp teeth, however, because they can cut into the hair and cause damage.) Giving your child combs and brushes and teaching

her the proper way to wash her hair can instill good grooming habits that could last a lifetime.

However, even the most well cared-for child may one day
come home from school or day care with an unwelcome
guest: lice. Head lice infestation, in fact, affects more school-
age children than any other communicable disease. It is
caused when these tiny brown parasitic insects take up residence in the scalp, feeding on the child's blood, laying eggs
(or "nits"), and causing intense itching of the scalp. They can
spread from child to child through close contact or through
hats, combs, or brushes that are shared. If you suspect your
child has lice, use a comb to separate the hair carefully and
see if you can spot any of the yellowish-white nits on the
hair, especially at the nape of the neck, behind the ears, and
at the crown of the head. Using a magnifying glass may help.
Once you spot the nits, call your pediatrician to see if he or
she can recommend one of the many pesticidal shampoos
that are available to treat lice. After washing your child's hair,
you will have to pick through the hair with a comb to remove the dead—and any surviving—insects and nits in the
hair. Sometimes a second shampoo treatment is recommended for seven to ten days later to ensure complete removal of any residual eggs that might have hatched. In addition, you will need to wash any clothing or linens that your
child has used over the last several days in very hot water to
kill any lice that may have gotten on them. You should also
check other family members to ensure that transmission of
the lice hasn't already occurred, and notify your child's
teacher to ensure that the other children in the classroom are
also checked and, if necessary, treated for the condition.
Chances are a few other children in your child's class have
lice too; the infestation is highly contagious.

Adolescence

The fact that the skin's sebaceous glands increase in size and
produce more oil during adolescence affects the appearance

not only of skin but also of hair. Hair that used to stay clean and bouncy when shampooed as little as once a week may now need to be washed daily because the increased oils in the scalp cause it to look "greasy" sooner. Very active, athletic teens may need to wash their hair as often as twice a day because exercise can raise the body's temperature, causing even more oil to be produced in the oil glands. Oily hair that isn't washed frequently enough could exacerbate acne by increasing the amount of oil on the skin.

Hormonal stimulation at puberty also causes another startling change: vellus hairs on certain parts of the body develop into terminal hairs. In girls this happens particularly in the legs, underarms, and genital area. Some girls also notice hair in typically "male" areas—the upper lip, chin, and even on the abdomen and chest. In most cases such distribution of hairs is due to heredity and is not a medical concern. But most girls are at least somewhat disconcerted by this sprouting of body hair, and reassurance that these body changes are perfectly normal can be vital to a girl's self-esteem and self-image. This is the age when girls begin experimenting with hair-removal techniques, and parental guidance in this regard can help to prevent hair-removal disasters such as irritant reactions and loss of hair from places where they don't want it (caused, for example, by misplaced depilatories). (For information on hirsutism and hair-removal techniques, see Chapter 9, pages 149–158.)

Signs of fad diets and eating disorders, fairly common in the teen years, can also show up in hair in the form of dry, brittle, damaged hair. Of course, such symptoms are also common in young women who overstyle their hair. But when hair looks unusually dry and brittle or if it begins to fall out—and especially if these symptoms are accompanied by other body symptoms such as weight loss and menstrual irregularity—a visit to the doctor is warranted.

Twenties to Forties: The Reproductive Years

At the age of twenty, according to some research, a woman's hair is the thickest it will ever be. Hair gradually thins over the next fifty years or so, until by age seventy most women notice that their hair is much finer and softer than it was in their youth. That pattern of hair thinning changes, however, when a woman becomes pregnant. Hair, like skin and nails, is controlled to a great extent by the body's hormonal production. Estrogen is thought to encourage hair growth and thickness, and the body produces large amounts of estrogen during pregnancy. For this reason many women enjoy a fullness in their hair during pregnancy that is unequaled at any other time in their lives. About three months after a woman delivers her baby, however, she may notice larger amounts of hair in her brush than usual. It is thought that this postpartum hair loss is caused by a decrease in estrogen production after pregnancy. Some doctors also believe that the extreme stress of childbirth may "turn off" certain hair follicles, causing the hairs to fall out about three months later. Whatever the cause, hair rarely becomes noticeably thinner than it was before pregnancy, and the accelerated hair loss generally diminishes by about six months after delivery.

Of course, any woman in this age group who experiences sudden, noticeable hair loss should consult her physician. This could signal an underlying sickness or hormonal condition that may need treatment. Hair loss that is also accompanied by adult acne, menstrual irregularities, and/or infertility problems is especially likely to signal a hormonal dysfunction.

Most Caucasian women also begin to notice their first gray hairs after they enter their thirties (and some women notice these hairs in their twenties or even their teens). By age thirty, about 25 percent of all Caucasian women have noticeably graying hair. Interestingly, black women tend to go gray at a later age, forty-four on average. Yet surprisingly, less than one-third of women ever become completely white-haired (fair-haired women are more likely to). A handful of people never get any gray hairs at all. Your likelihood of turning gray is dependent primarily on your heredity. If your parents turned gray at an early age, you are likely to also. And if you are lucky enough to be among the handful of people whose parents kept their pigmented locks into old age, you probably will never go gray either.

As mentioned earlier in this chapter, gray hair is caused by the absence of pigment in the hair shaft. Individual strands may appear grayish at first as the pigment in the hair shaft lessens, but eventually those strands will most likely turn to white. Even when they do, however, when mixed together with pigmented strands of hair, they will most likely take on the look of gray. Although many women enjoy the change of their hair from dark to gray, many women during this age also begin to experiment with hair color. Today there are more options in hair color than ever before. (For more information on this subject, see Chapter 8.)

Fifty-Plus

By the time a woman has passed through menopause, the changes in her hair may be rather dramatic. Her hair may be substantially thinner than it was in her youth, and most likely it is grayer. In fact, close to 50 percent of women regularly color their hair by the time they enter their forties and fifties. Interestingly, this number declines slightly after age sixty, when many women accept and even grow to like their lighter locks. Skin pigment usually has also lightened slightly by this time, making it a better complement to gray hair.

As mentioned, estrogen production has a strong influence on hair growth and thickness. After menopause the body's production of estrogen declines dramatically, and the body's circulating androgens—male hormones—may take on a more dominant role in the body. Androgens are thought to have negative effects on hair diameter. For these reasons many postmenopausal women struggle with thinning hair. There is some anecdotal evidence that estrogen replacement therapy may improve hair thickness in postmenopausal women, but there is scant scientific evidence to support these observations. (For more information on hair loss, see Chapter 9.)

The increased influence of androgens in postmenopausal women also may cause sprouting of hairs in places a woman has never had them before—on the chin, for example, or above the lip. Postmenopausal women who notice these problems may want to look into electrolysis, which is well suited for removing most excess facial hair. Happily, some women notice a lessening of hair on their legs and find that they need to shave their legs less frequently as they age past menopause.

One of the wonderful things about hair is that making a small change in hairstyle or color can cause a major change in your appearance, and few women go through life without at least experimenting with a different color or with permanent waves or straightening procedures. Yet most of us probably don't know just how these processes work. You will begin to find out by turning the page.

CHAPTER 8

Changing Your Hair's Color or Texture

One out of every three American women colors her hair. Most of us do so either to cover hair that is turning gray or to lighten our natural hair color. In addition, it's been estimated that every day 250,000 women worldwide perm their hair. Many more opt for temporary changes in hair's texture through use of hot or cold rollers, curling irons, and other techniques. As widespread as the use of hair coloring and perming products is, relatively few women understand exactly how they work. This chapter will offer some explanations.

Changing Your Hair's Color

The idea of changing one's natural hair color is hardly new, although our methods have gotten much more sophisticated over the years. Cleopatra and her contemporaries in Egypt used henna rinses on their hair. Roman women during Julius Caesar's reign used a mixture of fat and ashes to lighten their hair to match the blond hair of English women that Caesar had taken captive. And those gorgeous red and golden highlights seen in the hair of the women Titian painted in the sixteenth century were, more often than not, achieved by using alkaline solutions on the hair and then exposing the hair to hours of sunlight.

Today's Choices in Hair Color

Today there are five types of hair color that are used most commonly: temporary, progressive, vegetable, semi-permanent, and permanent. Each has its own advantages and disadvantages.

Temporary Hair Color

Lasting through only one shampoo, temporary hair-coloring products tend to be the gentlest and safest—they don't contain ammonia or peroxide, and irritant and allergic reactions are rare. The dyes, which have such names as FD&C Red No. 4 and D&C Yellow No. 10, are many of the same dyes used in textiles. They have a high molecular weight that cannot penetrate into the hair shaft. Consequently, the hair shaft is simply coated with color, which washes out easily. Temporary colors can darken the hair or add streaks of color but cannot lighten the hair. Many women use temporary hair colors as an introduction to hair color and a chance to experiment with new shades.

Progressive Hair Color

The most well-known brand of progressive hair color is Grecian Formula. This type of product uses a metallic dye (usually lead acetate) that deposits a colorless water-soluble lead salt on the hair that reacts with the air to form lead oxide and lead sulfide, which are brown shades. The color produced by these dyes can look artificial and "flat," according to some professional colorists, and hair that is treated with a metallic dye cannot be changed with permanent colors or waves until the color is either chemically removed or the colored hair grows out.

Semi-Permanent Hair Color

Although actually a contradiction in terms, semi-permanent hair color is hair color that can be washed away in about six shampoos. It's not quite temporary but not quite permanent. (Recently Clairol introduced what they call "long-lasting semi-permanent haircolor," which contains an alkaline ammonia substitute that enables the color to last longer than most semi-permanent hair colors.) These dyes often come in the convenient form of "shampoo-in" hair color, meaning that the dyes are in a detergent base. The dyes are of low molecular weight and can therefore penetrate the hair cuticle easily and get into the hair cortex. Most semi-permanent hair colors contain several different dyes to give a more natural-looking color. The dyes have long chemical names such as 2-nitro-p-phenylenediamine and HC Blue No. 2. Semi-permanent hair colors come with instructions for doing a patch test on the skin twenty-four hours before use because this kind of hair color can cause allergic reactions in a small number of women.

Vegetable Dyes

Vegetable dyes coat the hair shaft with color. By far the most widely used vegetable dye is henna. Henna is derived from the *Lawsonia* shrub, which grows naturally in North Africa, India, and Sri Lanka. Once synonymous with red, henna now is available in an impressive palette from raven black to honey blond because manufacturers today use all parts of the plant to attain different shades. In addition, some professional colorists mix henna with other vegetable tints such as blueberry, raspberry, and walnut to add dimension to dark hair, and camomile and curry to add different tones to light hair.

Unlike other at-home hair colors, which come in neat kits and are relatively easy to apply, henna can be tedious and time-consuming. The henna powder must first be steeped in boiling water, then applied to the hair as a paste and covered with aluminum foil or a plastic bag. You then need to sit under a dryer or out in the hot sun for a minimum of thirty minutes or as long as two hours while the henna penetrates. (The longer you wait, the more intense the color will be.)

Because henna coats the hair shaft and "closes" the cuticle layer of the hair, the hair reflects light more evenly and so looks shinier after a henna treatment. Its use over many centuries also gives it a virtually flawless safety record. But henna does have limitations: repeated applications can result in "overhenna," in which the hair takes on unpleasant orange colors and/or feels tacky or weighed down. Because it coats the hair shaft, permanent hair color and permanent waves do not take well on henna-treated hair. And henna cannot lighten hair but only add shades of deeper colors.

Permanent Hair Color

Although both metallic and vegetable dyes can have permanent effects on hair, when most people refer to permanent hair color they are speaking of colors that occur because of an oxidation reaction within the hair. These are the only types of color that can either darken or lighten the hair. Such procedures as frosting, highlighting, and one- and two-step bleaching fall into this category, although technically these may involve only the removal of natural color and not always the addition of artificial color. Still, the changes are permanent.

About 70 percent of women who use hair color choose this type of permanent color. In permanent hair coloring, colorless dye-forming materials in an alkaline base (usually ammonia) are mixed, just prior to application, with a developer. The developer contains hydrogen peroxide (an acid). The alkaline substance when mixed with peroxide swells the hair shaft, allowing the tiny dye particles to penetrate into the cortex of the hair. Those colorless particles then react with the oxygen produced by the hydrogen peroxide, and they begin to combine with one another to produce the desired color. When they combine, their molecular weight increases, making them too large to escape out of the cortex of the hair and ensuring that the new color will be permanent. In addition to producing the oxygen necessary for this chemical reaction to occur, hydrogen peroxide also has the unique ability to lift color, bleaching the natural melanin in the hair shaft; it is hydrogen peroxide that enables permanent hair color products to lighten hair.

However, the hydrogen peroxide and ammonia in most shampoo-in hair colors can lift the hair's color by only one or two shades. So if your natural hair color is medium brown, you may be able to lighten your hair to a dark blond, but you won't be able to go to a platinum blond. That dramatic a change requires a two-step process (sometimes called a double process). First the natural pigment in the hair is pre-lightened using hydrogen peroxide and a "booster" ingredient that is a stronger ammonia solution, usually ammonium persulfate. Then the desired color is added back into the hair by applying a toner that contains either semi-permanent or permanent hair colors.

Many experts advise against double-process color because the aggressive chemicals can cause breakage and damage to the hair if not applied correctly and because the color change can be so dramatic that touch-ups at the roots of the hair have to be done more frequently, adding to the cost and the inconvenience of the procedure. Finally, double-processed hair often isn't flattering to complexions that were meant to be complemented by hair a totally different color.

Women with gray hair may have better success with two-step coloring than women whose hair is fully pigmented. Since gray hair is really just white (depigmented) hair mixed in with darker strands, all that has to be bleached are the strands that still have color.

Ten Tips for Better Hair Color

1. Choose the right color for you. According to Clairol research, the most common mistake that women make is choosing a semi-permanent or permanent hair color that is too dark. The best idea: choose a color that is one shade lighter than you think you want, particularly if you are using color to cover hair that is just starting to

turn gray. Since the product will darken not only your gray hair but the pigmented hair as well, your hair will likely have a darker overall appearance than you planned. And it's usually easier to correct a too light color than a too dark color. The pictures of models on the hair color packages can give you some sense of what the color will look like, but they are no guarantee; the color you end up with depends in part on the color you start out with.

2. Do a patch test one day before each and every time you color your hair. Most at-home kits come with step-by-step guidelines for how to do one of these simple tests, which will tell you whether or not you have developed an allergy to the product. If you have, doing a patch test ahead of time could prevent an allover allergic reaction.

3. If you are lightening your hair, stay within one or two shades of your natural hair color. This slight change will allow for the most natural-looking color and will minimize the line of demarcation at the roots of the hair as your natural color grows in, making for less frequent touch-ups.

4. If you're coloring to cover gray, realize that semi-permanent colors work best just when you are beginning to turn gray. Once your hair is more than 50 percent gray, you will have to switch to a permanent color for adequate coverage and natural-looking color.

5. Start out slowly. If you're a bit timid about making a color change, start with semi-permanent color or opt for subtle highlights rather than allover color. The change will be easy to correct if necessary, and you won't be a slave to "grow-out."

6. Use any at-home product in a well-ventilated room. Many have strong odors that some women consider unpleasant.

7. Choose the right shampoo and conditioner for your newly colored hair (see pages 163–167.) And use a deep

conditioner once a week or so on your hair to minimize damage.

8. Avoid excessive exposure to sun, salt, and chlorine after you have colored your hair. All of these elements can cause discoloration and further damage to your hair.

9. If you want to perm and color your hair, perm your hair first and wait one or two weeks before coloring; permanent wave chemicals can lighten hair further.

10. When in doubt, consult a professional colorist. This is especially important for color corrections; if you've already made one mistake, it's best not to make any more.

Correcting Color Disasters

The reason so many women begin coloring their hair with semi-permanent or temporary colors is that they know that nothing looks worse than a bad color job. Using hair color takes some practice and often learning from a few mistakes, and because semi-permanent and temporary colors wash out within a few shampoos, those mistakes can be short-lived.

Many mistakes with permanent hair color can be avoided by first doing a strand test—taking a few strands of hair and applying the hair color and waiting to see what the color will be and how long it takes to develop. Then, if the color is what you want, the same timing can be used for optimal color of all of your hair. Many professional hairdressers routinely do such strand tests. When using at-home hair color, carefully read all the instructions first and then follow them exactly to minimize color disasters.

What can you do if you do everything right and the color still comes out wrong? There are some solutions:

• If you used either a progressive hair color or a vegetable dye and the color came out too dark or flat, there are products on the market (Clairol's Metalex is one) designed to remove the coat of color that these types of hair color deposit on hair. Certain shampoos that are designed to remove unwanted color (such as Redken's Cleansing Creme or Clairol's "Uncolor") may also work.

- If you used a permanent hair color and your color came out too dark, a professional hair colorist may be able to apply highlights to counteract the darker color and give the hair some dimension. Some professional colorists may also try a very diluted solution of oil bleach, shampoo, and water to lighten the color a bit. If you can stand to wait, it might be best to let the color grow out for about two months and then apply a color one shade lighter than your previous hair color only to the roots.

- If you used a semi-permanent color to cover gray and your hair came out uneven in color, wash it at least once a day until the semi-permanent color is removed, then try using a permanent hair color, choosing a color one or two shades lighter than what you think you want. The long-lasting semi-permanent colors can often bestow a flattering and natural look to graying hair; the hair that is still pigmented will take on darker tones, but the gray strands won't darken as much with the hair color and so will look like subtle highlights in the hair, an appealing effect.

- If your blond hair has taken on a greenish cast, the same products you can use for removing metallic or vegetable dyes should work in this case too. There are even shampoos designed to be used after swimming that contain chelating ingredients. They can remove the deposits of copper in the hair that caused the green to occur. (Contrary to popular belief, the green that results from swimming in chlorinated water is not from the chlorine in the pool but from the copper piping through which most pool water flows. The same thing can result if the piping in your home is copper.)

- If your hair looks too blond, a professional colorist may be able to add color back into your hair with "low lights" (strands of darker hair color woven throughout the hair) or another method. It is also a good idea to get your hair back into good condition with regular conditioning treatments and by giving it a good trim to remove the split ends that are likely to have resulted from use of harsh bleaching chemicals.

Is Hair Color Safe?

For many women safety is the most important concern relating to hair color. Even women who swear they will "never go gray" or "always be blond" may harbor fears about the effects of using hair color on their short- and long-term health. Health concerns about hair color generally fall into two categories: allergic and irritant local reactions to hair color, and long-term reactions that may affect overall health.

Allergic and irritant reactions to temporary hair colors are highly unusual because the dyes used in these products are mild and because they are so quickly washed out of the hair. About one in every 500,000 applications of permanent hair color will result in an allergic reaction, and while semi-permanent hair colors can also cause allergic reactions, the incidence is even lower. The reaction will usually consist of a red, sometimes blistering rash on the scalp and along the hairline of the face; the skin may be inflamed and feel itchy or burning. Women who do patch tests religiously are likely to avoid allergic reactions. Any woman who has what she thinks is an allergic reaction to a hair color should contact her dermatologist, who may prescribe medications to reduce inflammation and will likely suggest that she avoid using hair-coloring products in the future.

Some women may experience slight stinging and a warm sensation on their scalps when they apply permanent haircoloring products. These sensations are to be expected because the ammonia and peroxide in the products can be slightly caustic. These symptoms shouldn't be confused with those of a true allergy, which is an immune response in the skin.

When it comes to the long-term effects of hair color on a woman's health, the picture becomes a little foggy. In test tubes hair-coloring chemicals have been shown to damage DNA, and laboratory animals fed massive amounts of hair dye chemicals have developed cancer. The big question is whether or not the comparatively minuscule doses of hair color that are absorbed through one's scalp can have the same kinds of effects found in laboratory mice that have consumed massive doses of these chemicals orally? The consensus from most experts is probably not. In fact, no study has ever directly connected cancer or other diseases in humans with the use of hair color. One recent study from the National Cancer Institute found that women with certain types of lymphoma were 50 percent more likely to say they had dyed their hair sometime in their lives than people who didn't have cancer. But this study alone does not provide a solid link between hair-coloring products and lymphoma. Several large-scale studies have found no link between hair color use and breast cancer or bladder cancer.

If you believe there are risks to using hair color, Dr. Sheila Hoar Zahm, an epidemiologist at the National Cancer Institute, suggests that you can minimize your risks by following the advice below:

- Opt for semi-permanent colors or light-colored permanent hair colors; these have less of the worrisome chemicals than permanent colors that tint hair dark shades.

- Opt for highlighting or frosting rather than allover hair color; because these procedures are often done by pulling strands of hair through a plastic cap, little or none of the hair color comes in direct contact with the scalp.

- Wear plastic gloves when applying hair color to your scalp or someone else's hair to prevent absorption of the chemicals through the skin of your hands.

- Don't have your hair colored during the first trimester of pregnancy. Although there is no evidence that hair color can have any effects on a developing fetus, many obstetricians recommend avoiding hair coloring during these first three months when the baby's major development takes place—just to be on the safe side. If you do want to color your hair during pregnancy, consider using a highlighting procedure.

Changing Your Hair's Texture

As women, it seems, we are never satisfied with our hair. Women with curly or kinky hair long for soft, shiny, straight locks. Women with straight hair often would give anything for their hair to have the body and movability of curls.

Your hair's "texture" is a combination of two factors: its diameter (whether it's coarse, fine, or in between) and its basic shape (straight, wavy, or curly). We tend to think of diameter as varying depending on one's race and heredity. Darker-skinned individuals (blacks, Asians, and American Indians) tend to have coarser hair than fair-skinned women (of northern European descent, for example). But hair can vary among people with similar backgrounds, and strands of hair can even vary on the same person. Looked at under a microscope, the diameter of all hair is represented by a circular shape. The outline of the circle is the hair's cuticle layer, while the interior of the circle is the hair's flexible cortex. In fine hair the diameter—comprised of the hair's cortex—is less than in coarse hair, making the cuticle layer proportionately greater. This difference may account for the reason that fine hair often doesn't hold a set as well as coarse hair; the cuticle layer is hard and resistant compared to the more flexible cortex, and that cuticle layer simply resists being reshaped by rollers.

Hair's natural shape, like its diameter, also depends on a woman's genetic background. As a rule, blacks tend to have curly, even "kinky" hair, and Asian women tend to have very straight hair, while the hair of Caucasian women can vary greatly from one extreme to the other. Again, hair curliness can differ among women of the same race. By looking at cross-sections of hair under microscopes, hair researchers have discovered that curly hair looks the most elliptical microscopically, while straight hair appears as a circle. Interestingly, straight hair is much easier to comb when dry, and curly hair is much easier to comb when wet (and the water has softened the curl slightly).

Hair shape can be temporarily changed by softening the hair with water and/or a setting lotion and then reshaping it around rollers. Heat can also be used to reshape hair temporarily around a curling iron or curlers. Once hair is set, hairspray, which produces bonds between hair strands, increasing the hold of the set, can make a hairstyle stay put. However, once the hair is exposed to water—either during bathing or in excessive humidity—the new hair shape immediately is lost.

How Does a Perm Work?

You can change your hair's shape permanently (or at least until the hair grows in) with the use of permanent wave solutions. As we have discussed earlier, hair is made of protein molecules, which are joined together by chemical bonds known as disulfide bonds to form the hair shaft. The shape of your hair depends on the particular configuration of the protein molecules to the disulfide bonds on your hair shaft. For example, in straight hair the protein molecules and the disulfide bonds are parallel to each other on the hair shaft; in curly hair the bonds and the protein molecules are at right angles to each other.

Permanent waves work by breaking down these disulfide bonds and then reforming them in the shape of the rods used in the hair. Perms generally involve three steps:

1. In the first step a perming solution is applied to break down the disulfide bonds; the lotion swells the hair's

cuticle layer and penetrates through to the cortex of the hair.

2. In the next step the hair is wrapped around rods or other objects that determine the new shape of the hair. The smaller the rod, the tighter the curl. (Today many top stylists wrap hair around objects ranging from tongue depressors to star shapes to get unique looks from a perm.) Often at this point the hair is exposed to heat, which can speed up the lotion's breakdown of the disulfide bonds; the lotion is then rinsed off thoroughly and the hair is blotted dry.

3. In the final step a neutralizer is applied to the hair. This lotion penetrates into the cortex and forces the disulfide bonds to relink in the shape suggested by the rods. Hair is rinsed and then unwrapped.

Types of Perms

Early perms used harsh chemicals that damaged hair and sometimes even caused hair loss. Today the amount of damage a permanent does to hair has been greatly reduced, and there are more types of perms than ever before to choose among. Here are some definitions of the most commonly used permanent waves.

Alkaline perms are probably the most commonly used salon perm. They are best used on virgin hair because they tend to be the most aggressive type of perm and so can cause the most damage to the hair. They produce the tightest, longest-lasting results. They have a pH of 9 or more, and in most alkaline perms, the active ingredient is ammonium thioglycolate.

Acid perms are "acid" only in comparison to alkaline perms, as their pH is more neutral, about 6–7. The active ingredient in these perms is usually glyceryl monothioglycolate, a less aggressive chemical than that used in alkaline perms. Acid perms are less damaging to hair and thus can often be used on color-treated hair. The curls they produce are likely to be softer and possibly not as long lasting as those of alkaline perms.

Bisulfite perms carry the least risk of damage of all of the perms. Sodium bisulfite is used most commonly in at-home perm products to reduce the risk of damage to the hair. The curl it produces is probably the loosest and shortest-lived. They can be used on color-treated hair, although in some cases the sodium bisulfite may lighten the hair slightly.

In addition to these three basic types of perms, there are many newer perms that have special features, including conditioning ingredients that penetrate into the hair cortex, minimizing damage to the hair, and ingredients that automatically stop the breakdown of the disulfide bonds, thus preventing damage (these are found in so-called self-timing perms).

Tips on Getting the Best Results

Next to bad hair color, few things look as terrible as bad perms; they can make you look like you just stuck your finger in an electric socket. But there are steps you can take before and after your perm to minimize problems and maximize your results.

Before You Perm . . .

- Condition your hair with a deep conditioner at least once a week for at least two weeks.

- Cut off any dry, split ends. If you don't, they will give your hair a "frizzy" look after perming.

- Don't color your hair right before perming. Most permanent wave chemicals lighten your hair slightly, and the color you had may no longer be the same color after a perm.

- Choose the right perm for your hair. Your hair doesn't have to be chemically treated to be damaged and to be a poor candidate for an alkaline perm. Excess sun exposure and overzealous styling (especially with heated styling tools) can also cause damage. Discuss the porosity, elasticity, length, and diameter of your hair with your stylist before having your hair permed.

- Consider perming only parts of your hair. If you want lift at the top of your hair, a root perm may be enough. If you want waves at the end, roll just the ends and apply solution to them. (Some experts suggest that an easy way to do this is to separate the hair into pigtails and then perm only the parts outside the pigtail holder.) Some women perm only the underlayers of their hair to add body and leave the top layers straight to reflect shine. Other women prefer to perm only the very top layer of their hair. Just as highlighting hair causes less damage than allover color, these partial perms are also less damaging than allover perms.

- Get a professional perm—at least the first time you do it. Thereafter you can discuss perming options with your stylist. If you do choose to do your perms at home, try to get a dexterous friend to help you roll the hair on the rods. It's extremely difficult to do a good job rolling your whole head of hair yourself. (Make sure to roll hair in small sections, so that the lotion is able to penetrate the hair on the rods completely.)

After the Perm . . .

- Wait forty-eight to seventy-two hours before washing your hair. This is important; it may take that long for all of the bonds to be re-formed completely.

- Use shampoos and conditioners specifically formulated for use on permed hair. (These usually have a low pH to complement the slightly higher pH of the hair after being permed.)

- Be gentle when combing and brushing your hair to prevent further damage.

- Avoid sun and excessive perspiration; both can further damage your hair.

- Talk to your stylist about new ways to style your "new" hair. Your old techniques and styling products may no longer work well.

- Have frequent trims; letting your hair grow too long after a perm can cause the waves to droop.

Straightening Hair

The idea behind straightening excessively curly or kinky hair is the same as that for curling straight hair: the protein bonds in the hair are changed to alter the shape of the hair into a desired style. Straightening can be done temporarily with waving lotions or heat, or permanently (until new hair grows in) with chemical straightening lotions and relaxants. No straightening procedure is recommended on hair that has previously been treated with a vegetable dye or a metallic dye. And if you have had any chemical process on your hair, consult your hairstylist before attempting to relax or straighten your hair with hot combs or chemical procedures.

Pomades

When pomades are combed through hair, their heavy oils weigh down the hair, making it appear a bit straighter but also very slick and greasy. The results are temporary; hair becomes curly again when the pomade is shampooed out. This method of hair straightening is not recommended for women with acne-prone skin. In a condition known as pomade acne, blemishes arise along the hairline of the face after exposure of the skin to an oily pomade, which can clog pores.

Hot Combs

One common method of straightening very curly hair is with a hot comb. Usually warm oil is applied to the hair first, and then the heated metal comb is pulled through the hair, changing the hair's protein bonds through the heat and stretching the hair into a straighter shape. Women who opt for this method run the risk of singeing their hair if the oil or the comb is too hot or burning their scalp and facial and neck skin if the hot oil drips into those areas. Therefore extreme caution must be exercised when using a hot comb to straighten hair. After the initial relaxing of the hair, many women then roll their hair in curlers and expose it to more heat. Obviously, all of this heat causes some breakage of the hair, and both daily conditioners and weekly intensive conditioners are usually recommended. Generally the hot comb method of relaxing hair lasts just until the next shampoo.

Chemical Relaxers

For turning moderately curly hair into wavy hair (not into completely straight hair), many experts recommend curly perms, which contain the same active ingredients as permanent waves for straight hair—thioglycolates (in salon perms) and bisulfites (in at-home perms). Before using curly perms, it's important to do a strand test to determine exactly the length of time you should leave the product on the hair shaft before rinsing and neutralizing the hair. A patch test should also be done twenty-four hours before applying the product to the hair to minimize the risk of allergy to the product. Most products come with detailed instructions on how to do each of these tests.

Before a curly perm lotion is used, the hair should be thoroughly washed, towel-dried, and combed. Straightening lotion is then applied over all of the hair and combed through. The hair is wrapped in plastic and the solution is allowed to penetrate for ten to twenty minutes (or as long as was necessary in the strand test). Next, the plastic is removed and the hair is combed through again. The hair is then rinsed and towel-dried, and a neutralizing lotion is applied, left on the hair for five minutes, and rinsed out. The hair is then set with rollers into the desired style. Frequent conditioning is recommended after a curly perm to keep the wave soft and manageable and to minimize damage to the hair.

Chemical Straighteners

To make very curly or kinky hair straight, stronger chemicals are required to break down the protein bonds in the hair. The most common ingredient in chemical straighteners is sodium hydroxide, a highly alkaline substance that can be very irritating to the scalp and damaging to the hair. For this reason women are often advised to apply a base of pomade on the scalp and hairline before applying the straightener to the hair. This oily layer protects the scalp from the irritating chemicals.

Unlike curly perms, which are applied to damp hair, chemical straighteners are applied to dry hair and combed through; the sodium hydroxide breaks down the hair's protein bonds, and the repeated combing encourages the hair to take a straighter shape. Once the hair looks straight, the straightener is rinsed out of the hair thoroughly, and a neutralizing solution is applied to re-form the hair bonds in the straighter style.

The riskiest part of using chemical straighteners containing sodium hydroxide comes when it's time to "touch up" the hair, about three or four months after the initial straightening, when a significant amount of the naturally curly hair has grown in. The straightener should be applied only to the new growth of the hair, which can be tricky to do. If the product does have contact with the previously straightened parts of the hair, that hair can become so severely damaged that it breaks off near or at the root, sometimes leaving small bald patches on the scalp. Although the hair will most likely grow back, living with the bald patches in the interim can be hard on one's self-image. For this reason most experts recommend that chemical straighteners be applied only by professional stylists who have a lot of experience using them.

Tips for More Successful Straightening

- Have your hair straightened professionally the first few times you do it (if not all of the time). You'll get a sense of what the procedure entails and tips on how best to do it if you then want to attempt hair straightening at home.

- Never use chemical straighteners, relaxants, or hot combs on hair if the scalp is already irritated; all of these procedures have the potential to irritate the scalp further.

- If a rash, sores, or persistent irritation of the scalp results from straightening the hair, see a dermatologist.

- Never straighten hair that has been previously colored yourself. The straightening won't work if the color was henna or a metallic dye. And if the hair was permanently colored, it is already damaged and may not withstand further damage from the straightening procedure.

- Do a strand test and a patch test each and every time you use a chemical straightener or relaxant because the timing of the product may be different once your hair has already been processed and because you can develop an allergy to one of these products at any time.

- Keep all chemicals related to straightening away from the eyes. Sodium hydroxide can be particularly damaging, even leading to blindness if it gets in the eyes.

- Treat straightened hair with tender loving care. Use conditioner religiously. Avoid rough combing and brushing, which can cause further hair breakage, and don't towel-dry your hair too vigorously after shampooing. Avoid excess sun exposure and perspiration, both of which can add to the damage to hair. Consult your stylist about the best hair products for your newly straightened hair.

CHAPTER 9

Solving Common Hair Problems

If, as is often said, a woman's hair is her "crowning glory," then it is no wonder that problems with our hair can be so upsetting. It's a rare woman who goes through life without some problems with head and/or body hair. Either she has too much hair (especially in places she doesn't want it, like above her lip or in the bikini area) or too little (on her head), or her hair is too oily or too dry, or she has dandruff or some other hair problem. This chapter will address these common problems and offer some solutions.

Hair Loss in Women

Every single day you lose an average of 50 to 125 hairs from your head. This loss is hardly perceptible, since most women have an average of 100,000 hairs on their heads; natural blonds have slightly more hair on average (although the individual hairs tend to be finer), and redheads have slightly less (although each hair tends to be coarse and thick). Hair follows a very predictable pattern of growing, resting, and shedding. The growing phase is known medically as the anagen phase, and at any one time 85 to 90 percent of hair is in this phase, causing hair to grow about one inch per month. The hair keeps growing for a period lasting from two to six years. When the hair growth ends, the hair shaft begins a two- to six-month period of resting (known medically as the telogen phase) and then shedding. The resting phase, in which the hair stops growing but does not yet fall out, accounts for about 11 percent of hair strands at any one time. And the shedding phase accounts for only about 4 percent of hair at any one time. Noticeable hair loss occurs when less hair than normal is in the growing phase, and more than normal is in the shedding phase.

The Causes of Hair Loss

About 25 percent of women will notice some hair thinning or loss by the time they reach their late thirties. By the time they pass through menopause, about 60 percent of women will experience some noticeable hair loss. Throughout our lives, temporary hair loss can be caused by many different factors.

Extreme stress can cause the body to focus its energies on maintaining and repairing vital body structures, and growing hair is not one of them. In many cases there is a three-month delay between the stressful event and the onset of hair loss. And after hair has stopped falling out, there may be another three-month delay before it begins to grow back. That stressful event may be physical (surgery, illness) or emotional (the death of a loved one, depression). Some doctors believe that the stress of delivering a baby is one reason that many women experience hair loss about three months after childbirth. Of course, hormonal changes are also thought to play a role in hair loss after pregnancy.

Dietary deficiencies, caused by fad diets and conditions such as anorexia (self-starvation), can produce hair loss in some women.

Medications, such as the chemotherapeutic agents used for treating cancer, antidepressants, blood pressure medications, and high doses of vitamin A, can also cause hair loss.

Hormonal changes brought about by pregnancy, birth control pills, and menopause are associated with hair loss. Estrogen is thought to encourage hair growth, and this hormone is produced in abundance during pregnancy and is provided in some birth control pills. During and after menopause and after pregnancy, estrogen production decreases, and hair often becomes thinner. (Some birth control pills are also formulated to have more androgen effects than estrogen effects, and this formulation may lead to hair loss in some women.)

When hair loss is caused by one of these factors, hair usually begins to grow again once the underlying problem is solved. But there are two types of hair loss that are longer lasting or even permanent. The less common of these two types is known as alopecia areata. This condition affects approximately 2.5 million Americans—men, women, and children—and is thought to be caused by an underlying problem in a person's autoimmune system. It usually occurs in one of three forms: small circular areas of hair loss (alopecia areata), complete loss of scalp hair (alopecia totalis), and complete loss of all body hair (alopecia universalis). There are various treatments for this condition, including corticosteroid drugs, ultraviolet therapy, and immunosuppressive medications. Some of these treatment approaches work in some people, but there is no cure for everybody. However, in many cases of alopecia areata, the hair spontaneously begins growing again.

A much more common type of hair loss is known as androgenetic alopecia, or female pattern baldness (or, in men, male pattern baldness). Female pattern baldness usually begins when a woman is about thirty (although it can happen as early as puberty) and begins to be noticeable at about age forty, but becomes particularly noticeable after menopause. This patterned hair loss affects about one-third of women (and about one-third of men) and is believed to be determined by a woman's genetic and hormonal makeup. (Contrary to popular myth, which says that hair loss tendency is passed down through a person's mother, both a mother and father can contribute to a child's likelihood to have androgenetic alopecia.)

Because the pattern tends to differ from that of men, hair loss in women has not been given the wide attention that balding in men has received. Women's hair loss tends to appear as overall thinning, sometimes of the entire scalp, sometimes of just the front third or half of the scalp, and it is usually fairly easy to disguise for a long time with clever styling, coloring, and perming. In contrast, men usually experience male pattern hair loss in the form of a receding hairline and/or loss of hair at the crown of the head.

Nobody knows just what causes pattern hair loss. It is thought that more and more hair follicles simply stop producing hairs and begin to shrink in size. Some researchers believe that the "male" hormones known as androgens (present in both men and women) have a role in shutting down the hair follicles. This may explain why postmenopausal women seem to have a worse problem with this type of hair loss; women in this age group produce less estrogen, which counteracts the effects of androgens. There is some anecdotal evidence, although no hard scientific data, that estrogen replacement therapy may thicken scalp hair in some postmenopausal women and may also minimize the unwanted body hair that sometimes sprouts up on a woman's chin, chest, and in other traditionally "masculine" areas after menopause.

Hair Loss Treatments

Rogaine. Until recently there was no good treatment for female pattern hair loss. But with FDA approval of the drug minoxidil (in the topical solution Rogaine) in August 1991, women now have a somewhat effective, if still imperfect, treatment for androgenetic alopecia. Rogaine is a clear, non-oily liquid that is applied to the scalp twice a day. It is estimated that 60 percent of women with mild to moderate hair loss experience a minimal to moderate regrowth after six to eight months of therapy with this drug. It is unclear just how Rogaine works. Some researchers have noted that the hair follicles seem to enlarge when Rogaine is applied to the scalp. Others theorize that the drug may increase blood flow to the scalp by dilating blood vessels. (Minoxidil was originally approved in 1979 as a drug to control high blood pressure.)

Use of Rogaine is a lifelong commitment; once a woman stops applying the product to her scalp, she can expect most, if not all, of the new hairs she has grown to be shed within a matter of months. The drug can also cause some side effects, including irritation, itchiness, and redness of the scalp, and potentially some long-term side effects that are, as yet, unknown. The drug is also expensive, costing an average of six hundred dollars per year.

Aldactone. Another drug that is currently being researched for treatment of female pattern hair loss is a diuretic called spironolactone (known by the trade name Aldactone). In one recent study women who were treated with spironolactone for one year stopped losing their hair, while women who were not treated with the drug continued to lose hair; when the daily dose of the drug was doubled, hair density actually increased. More research is needed to determine just how spironolactone might work to restore hair growth in women and to ascertain its safety. It is known to have some side effects, including heavy periods and menstrual irregularities in women who take it.

Hair transplants. Some women with female pattern hair loss may be candidates for hair transplantation. In this procedure grafts of hair and skin are taken from areas with healthy hair follicles and transplanted into balding areas. Until recently this was not considered as viable an option for women as it was for men. The fact that women's hair loss tended to be more diffuse and could occur all over the head, rather than just in certain areas, meant that finding really healthy areas from which to graft was more difficult. Recent refinements in hair-transplanting techniques, such as mini- and micro-grafting, have enabled dermatologic surgeons to transplant thinning hair more successfully. These types of grafts also produce a more natural-looking hairline, and there's less risk of scarring (although there is still some risk).

Transplantations can be costly however, as high as ten thousand dollars, and are dependent somewhat on the skill of the surgeon. Ask your dermatologist or doctor for a referral to a surgeon who has a lot of experience with transplants in your area. Or contact the American Hair Loss Council (100 Independence Place, Suite 207, Tyler, TX 75703; 1-800-274-8717); the American Academy of Facial Plastic and Reconstructive Surgery (1110 Vermont Avenue NW, Suite 220, Washington, DC 20005; 1-800-332-FACE); or the American Society for Dermatologic Surgery (1-800-441-2737).

Styling and conditioning. While it's impossible to prevent female pattern baldness, the appearance of thinning hair can be minimized with careful styling and by preventing hair breakage due to mechanical damage (from too-hot blow dryers and curling irons, overly aggressive combing and brushing, and overperming, for example). Black women seem to be particularly prone to what is known as traction alopecia, a condition in which hair falls out in patches because of the constant tension or twisting of certain hairstyles, such as cornrows; also, repeated applications of straightening and coloring chemicals can weaken the hair, causing its loss in some instances.

Regular conditioning of thinning hair can make it comb more easily, preventing breakage, and may even coat the hair slightly to make it appear a bit thicker. Do not be taken in, however, by promises on the labels of nonprescription hair growth products. Vitamins, scalp massages, special creams, and special shampoos will not stop your hair from falling out or cause more hair to grow in. They will probably cause only more loss—from your pocketbook.

Scalp Problems

Often the problems that we associate with our hair are really skin conditions of the scalp. Three of the most common problems are dandruff, seborrheic dermatitis, and psoriasis of the scalp. Here are the wheres, whats, and what-you-can-dos for each.

Dandruff, by far the most common scalp ailment, is a condition in which scales of white flaky or grayish waxy material (dead skin) are shed by the scalp and clump together with scalp oils. It is known by the medical term *seborrhea,* and it affects about 50 percent of all women at some point. Usually it is associated with dry skin of the scalp, although many factors can be involved, including a hereditary predisposition to dandruff, stress, sickness, changes in the seasons (it's more common in the cold winter months), and the use of oily hairstyling products that are not completely washed out of the hair.

Seborrheic dermatitis occurs more prominently in people with oily hair and skin. Symptoms include red or yellow thick, scaly, greasy crusts on the scalp and sometimes also on the face, eyelids, and eyebrows and behind the ears. It's thought that seborrheic dermatitis might be caused in part by an overproduction of yeast organisms in the scalp, which feed on the scalp oils. Seborrheic dermatitis often causes itching and inflammation of the scalp and in the most severe cases can result in scarring and even hair loss. (For information on other kinds of dermatitis, see Chapter 4, pages 55–57.)

Psoriasis is thought to be caused by the hyperproliferation of skin cells on the scalp (and other body parts—see Chapter 4, page 52). These excess skin cells result in large, red, scaly patches that may itch or sting, swell, and be inflamed. The problem can be chronic and is thought to be hereditary.

While currently there is no cure for any of these problems, the symptoms can usually be relieved or minimized through use of special therapeutic shampoos. Before buying a shampoo and "self-treating" your problem, however, you would be wise to see a dermatologist for an accurate diagnosis. Ordinary dandruff usually responds well to use of a shampoo containing zinc pyrithione or sulfur and/or salicylic acid or selenium sulfide. These ingredients help to slow down the cell turnover rate of the scalp, reducing scaling. For seborrheic dermatitis or psoriasis, the best shampoos are those that contain coal tar, which not only slows cell turnover but also reduces inflammation and redness. (If your hair is blond or gray, be careful to choose a coal tar shampoo designed not to discolor light-colored hair; some coal tar shampoos can leave a greenish tinge on gray or blond hair.) In some cases of seborrheic dermatitis, a doctor may also prescribe antifungal agents, and for psoriasis or seborrheic dermatitis, sometimes topical steroids to reduce scalp inflammation.

The following are some other steps you can take to minimize your risks of dandruff, seborrheic dermatitis, and psoriasis:

- Don't overmassage your scalp when using shampoo or styling products or when brushing.

- Avoid very hot showers; hot water may further dry out the scalp, increasing your risks of dandruff.

- If the air in your home or office is very dry, use a humidifier.

- Remove your hat at the first sign of scalp sweating or itching.

- Choose a hairbrush with soft, round bristles; sharp bristles may further irritate the scalp.

- Avoid overuse of heated styling appliances such as hair dryers, curling irons, and heated rollers. They can irritate the scalp, worsening symptoms.

Too Much of a Good Thing: Hirsutism

For all the work we devote to grooming the hair on our head, most women spend equal or more time removing hair from where they don't want it. In most women excess body hair (known to doctors by the medical term *hirsutism*) is not a medical concern; it is due to heredity or to hormonal changes that occur during puberty, pregnancy, and menopause, or it occurs as a side effect of taking certain medications. But in about 10 percent of women, hirsutism can signal a problem with the ovaries or adrenal gland, particularly when a woman also has other symptoms such as hair loss from the scalp, menstrual irregularities, and acne. These symptoms together merit a visit to your doctor for blood tests to ensure that your hormone levels are normal. If a hormonal imbalance is detected, often doctors can successfully treat the problem with hormonal therapy.

Once you have hair in unwanted spots, however, it's bound to stay there for a long time, if not forever. This doesn't mean you can never show your legs on the beach again. It just means you may want to try out a few different hair-removal techniques until you find the one that works best for you.

General Hair-Removal Tips

- Never remove hair the morning of a day that you plan to spend at the beach or pool. The skin is always more sensitive immediately after any hair-removal technique and will be more prone to irritation from sunlight, sunscreens, salt water, and chlorinated water. Instead, remove hair the night before.

- If skin swelling, redness, or irritation does result from hair removal, stop what you're doing until the irritation subsides (which may be several days). If the irritation persists beyond a few days or if it comes back each and every time you remove hair in that area, see your dermatologist.

- Be especially vigilant about shaving excess hair from your underarms. In addition to non-odor-producing eccrine sweat glands, which are all over your body, your underarms also house apocrine sweat glands, which contain bacteria that can produce an offensive body odor when allowed to proliferate. Underarm hair shelters that bacteria, making this odor more likely; removing hair from the underarms, then, not only makes them look more attractive but can minimize underarm odor.

- Don't use any of the following hair-removal techniques on stray hairs that sprout out of moles, inner nose, ears, perianal and vaginal regions. The safest way to reduce the appearance of hair in these areas is to cut it back with small manicure scissors.

- If ingrown hairs (in which the tip of the hair grows back into the skin, causing inflammation) result from any of the following hair-removal techniques, try flicking them out with a sterile pointed tweezer. But if you do not succeed after two or three tries, wait a day or two and try again. If you don't succeed again, see your dermatologist. Getting too aggressive with ingrown hair removal is sure to cause infection and inflammation, which could ultimately lead to a scar. A dermatologist is more skilled and experienced at this tricky problem and will likely remove the hair with little or no difficulty.

Options in Hair Removal

Shaving

Shaving is the quickest, easiest, and most popular method of hair removal in this country (even though the results are the most short-lived of any hair-removal method), so it's not surprising that there are some popular myths about what shaving can and cannot do. Many women believe, for example, that once an area has been shaved, the hair grows back darker and thicker. This is not true. Shaving cuts the hair off at the skin surface, making the hair blunt at the top, which can cause it to look thicker and darker. (In the process, shaving also removes the uppermost layer of your skin, acting as a natural exfoliant and making your skin appear smooth.) But if you were to let the hairs grow in half an inch or so, you'd see they were the same type of hair that you removed days ago. The age at which you begin to shave also has nothing to do with the amount of hair you will have in shaved areas or with how fast it will grow back or with its color or thickness; those characteristics are determined by heredity and your hormonal makeup.

Here are some tips on how to get the closest shave:

- To minimize the risk of nicking yourself, use an electric razor or choose a disposable with a built-in moisturizing strip; they provide easy glide for the razor to slip over the skin, for a closer, nick-free shave.

- Since hair can begin to grow back and be noticeable in as little as twelve hours, shave every day.

- Do not shave stray facial hairs; stubble may appear within a few hours and look obvious.

- Do not shave first thing in the morning. Your skin tends to be a little bit puffy, causing it to be more prone to cuts and lessening the closeness of the shave. Wait at least half an hour or so before shaving.

- If you use an electric razor, shave in a circular motion on dry skin.

- If you use a disposable razor, choose one with a twin blade. The first blade extends the hair, and the second cuts it off for a closer, less stubbly shave.

- Wet the skin thoroughly before shaving with a disposable razor, and apply soap and water or shaving cream. Use warm, not hot or cold, water to prevent irritating the skin yet allow the pores to expand, exposing more of the hairs for a closer shave. Don't shave if your skin has been exposed to fifteen minutes or more of steady water (as in a long soak in a tub). The skin will be too puffy, and not enough of the hair will be exposed for adequate hair removal.

• Shave in the opposite direction of hair growth for the smoothest look. However, if this leads to irritation and red bumps (especially likely in the bikini area), wait until the area heals, then shave in the direction of hair growth (toward the feet on the legs). Underarm hair often grows in many different directions, so you may have to shave up and down for complete hair removal.

• Soothe skin immediately after shaving by sprinkling the area with unscented powder or cornstarch.

• Change your razor after a maximum of five uses, and store it in a cool, dry spot between shaves. (Leaving it in the shower to get wet repeatedly may cause it to rust; never use a rusty razor.)

Depilatories

Depilatory lotions and creams contain a strong alkaline solution (usually hydrogen sulfide) that dissolves body hair at the skin surface, providing hair removal that lasts from two days up to one week. It's important to choose a product that is specifically targeted for the area of body hair you are going to remove. For example, depilatories intended for use on the legs tend to be more concentrated than those meant for use on the upper lip, which is more prone to irritation. Since the ingredients in depilatories can cause allergic or irritant reactions in some women, it's best to do a small patch test of a depilatory product before applying it to a larger area. To do this, apply a small amount of the product to a nickel-sized area of the skin on your forearm; leave it on the amount of time indicated in the directions on the package, then rinse it off and wait twenty-four hours. If redness, swelling, or a rashlike irritation occurs in that area, do not use the depilatory. If not, apply the depilatory according to directions.

Since some depilatories carry a strong odor, it's usually best to apply them in a well-ventilated room.

Tweezing and Plucking

Tweezing your hair manually or removing it with one of the electric "pluckers," which snap up hair via a mechanism of revolving coils or rubber band–like projections, essentially accomplishes the same thing: it pulls hair out of the skin from the root. The results last longer (from a few days to a week) than those of shaving, but because of potential damage to the hair follicle, ingrown hairs are more likely. Manual tweezing is best for small areas (such as the eyebrows) and stray hairs. Many cosmeticians recommend stainless steel tweezers with slanted points for easier grasping of the hair. Before you begin to tweeze an area, it's a good idea to apply an antibacterial lotion to the skin to reduce the risk of infection. When you are ready to tweeze, stand before a well-lighted mirror, pull the skin taut with one hand, squeeze the tweezers around the base of the hair, and pull in the direction that the hair grows (toward your hairline for hairs under the brows, toward your forehead for hairs between brows). It should come out easily. To shape your eyebrows, many makeup pros emphasize not doing too much too soon; begin by just pulling out the stray hairs that don't follow the dominant shape of the brow. Tweeze just enough hairs underneath the brows to give them some definition, but do not make them pencil thin; tweeze hairs between the brows to give a softer look to your whole face. Sterilize the tweezers between uses by swabbing them with alcohol and/or rinsing them under very hot water and drying them for storage.

Electric pluckers may be used on larger areas than tweezers but require more time, and some women complain that they cause considerable pain. However, the results can be silky smooth. Before using an electric plucker, wash the area and rub it gently with a facecloth or loofah to make the hairs stand more erect, minimizing the risks of ingrown hairs. Dry the skin gently with a towel. Pull the skin taut with one hand as you pluck with the other, moving the device over the skin in a circular motion.

Waxing

Waxing, like tweezing and plucking, removes hair by the root, and over several years of steady waxing, often enough damage is done to the hair root that the hair just stops growing in or grows in more softly, so that less frequent removal is necessary. In a waxing procedure, hot or cold wax is applied to the skin in the direction of hair growth. The hair becomes trapped in the sticky wax, which is then pulled off in one quick motion in the opposite direction of hair growth. In skilled hands, waxing can be done quickly and cause only momentary stinging. But even in the most experienced hands, waxing involves a fairly high risk of ingrown hairs.

Most women prefer to have waxing performed professionally at least for the first few times to see if they can withstand the pain and if the results are worth the effort. But after a few sessions at the skin salon, you may be ready to try it on your own. Here are some suggestions.

• Remember that hot wax generally works better than cold to grip the hairs, providing more thorough removal. Test the temperature of the wax on the inside of your palm before applying it to the skin for hair removal, to prevent burns. (The wax should be no hotter than candle wax.)

• Wait until the hair is at least one-quarter inch long before applying wax; any shorter, and the wax won't be able to grip the hair for removal.

• Make sure the skin in the area is totally dry because the wax—hot or cold—won't work on damp skin. Sometimes applying talc or cornstarch before the wax is recommended for drying the skin.

• Don't wax your skin during the week before your menstrual period is due if you are at all prone to premenstrual symptoms. Many estheticians claim that the increased puffiness of the skin at this time can interfere with the results, and some women are less tolerant of the pain caused by waxing at this time of the month.

- Try waxing your lower legs first, since they are among the least sensitive areas that often need hair removal. If you can take the sting on your legs and are successful at removal, you may want to move up to your thighs and bikini area if you need hair removal in these places.

- Apply the wax in small strips, which are easier to remove.

- If you're using hot wax, wait until it has hardened completely before removal. Pick up just a small corner first to give yourself a good piece for gripping. Then, pulling the skin taut with your other hand, pull off the wax in the opposite direction of hair growth in one swift, strong movement.

- Your skin will sting momentarily; to lessen the sting, apply pressure to the area with your hand immediately after removing the wax.

- Don't wax any area more than once in one time. You'll only increase your risk of irritation.

- Soothe skin after waxing by applying a fragrance-free moisturizer.

Electrolysis

Electrolysis is the only way to remove hair permanently. An electrical current is transmitted to the hair root through a fine wire needle or probe that is inserted into the skin pore. The hair root is destroyed, and the hair is then easily removed with tweezers. Only about 60 percent of the hair in an area is destroyed in an initial electrolysis treatment, so that sometimes three or four treatments are needed for complete hair removal of an area. The process can be painful and somewhat tedious and for that reason is most suitable for small areas of hair removal, such as the chin, upper lip, and stray hairs in the bikini area. Slight redness and swelling immediately after electrolysis are common symptoms and usually go away within an hour. Occasionally small scabs can also appear two to four days after treatment; they should be left alone and will disappear on their own within a few days. Applying an antibiotic cream to the area can enhance the healing process. Avoid applying makeup to the skin for about one day after electrolysis, and avoid sunlight for several days.

Just how well electrolysis will work for you and how painful it will feel will depend in large part on the skill of the electrologist you see. If possible, make sure that your electrologist is licensed by your state (not all states require licensing), and ask your dermatologist for a reference. Ask if the electrologist is certified by the International Board of Electrology (CPE) or the National Commission for Electrology (CCE); these degrees mean that the electrologist was graduated from a recognized school of electrolysis, has had at least one year's clinical experience, has passed a certification exam, and is participating in continuing education to maintain certification. Also make sure that the electrologist and his or her establishment follow safe sterilization procedures: probes should be sterilized either in a dry heat oven or an autoclave, or disposable needles should be used once and discarded; the electrologist should wear disposable gloves during treatment; all towels and table linens should be changed and sanitized between clients; skin areas with open lesions or visible irritation should not be treated. Maintaining these standards is important to reduce the risks of spreading infection from client to client.

Don't attempt to do electrolysis on yourself using one of the often-advertised at-home electrolysis machines. Few untrained people have the skill to insert the probe into the pore correctly, and the result could be scarring and pitting of your skin.

If you are taking any medications, have any chronic conditions (such as diabetes), or have a history of enlarged scars (such as keloids), consult your physician before having electrolysis performed on your skin. You may not be a good candidate for this procedure.

CHAPTER 10

Drugstore Survival Guide for Your Hair

It may be difficult to believe, but before 1930, when Breck shampoo hit the market, shampoos as we know them today didn't exist. Women used bar soap or soaplike combinations of sodium hydroxide (lye) and plant or animal oil to wash their hair. Although soap provided a thorough cleanser for the hair, it also stripped away the hair's natural oils, making it dry and unmanageable, and left a dull film on the hair shaft.

Choosing and Using a Shampoo

Today we have hundreds of shampoos to choose from, ranging from those with exotic scents to those that promise to "nourish" the hair to those that offer extra shine, body, bounce, or protection. Despite the dizzying array of new products on the market, the basic dilemma of making a shampoo has always remained constant: a shampoo has to offer thorough cleansing to the hair but still be gentle enough to keep hair well moisturized and soft. This balancing act can be successfully accomplished by combining just the right ingredients in just the right amounts. There are some categories of ingredients that appear in all shampoos, and then there are ingredients that are added to give a shampoo specific qualities. And there might be some ingredients that are added just "for show." Learning how to read a shampoo label is one step toward becoming a smart consumer and will help you to choose the right shampoo for your hair.

What's in a Shampoo?

All shampoos have as their base the same two ingredients: detergent and water. The detergent is usually listed on the ingredient label as a "sulfate," often lauryl sulfate or laureth sulfate. (Because the sulfate will sting if it gets in the eyes, in baby shampoos it is often replaced by a cleansing agent that won't sting if it drifts down into the eye area; cocampho-carboxy propionate is a common one. These "amphoteric" detergents don't remove oil and dirt as thoroughly as sulfate detergents do, but since most children don't have oily hair, they don't need as thorough cleansing as adults.) The detergent is responsible not only for cleansing the hair but for bestowing some of the rich lather that some women find so pleasing. Beyond these two basic ingredients, most shampoos also contain one or more of the following types of ingredients.

Thickening agents. These ingredients thicken the consistency of the shampoo, making it easier to apply and helping the shampoo form a lather more readily. Salts, cellulose derivatives, and substances whose names end in -amide (such as lauramide or cocamide) are among the most common thickening agents used in shampoos.

Conditioning ingredients. These are designed to add some moisture back into the hair and to fill in the gaps on the hair's roughened cuticle caused by excessive use of heated styling tools, chemicals, and sun exposure. Natural plant oils (such as wheat germ oil, jojoba oil, coconut oil, and avocado oil), lanolin derivatives, proteins, carbohydrates and sugars, and synthetic ingredients such as silicones and polymers, all can provide conditioning qualities in a shampoo. Conditioning ingredients can also add shine to the hair by coating the hair shaft and allowing the hair cuticle to lie flat, making it better able to reflect light.

Preservatives. Anything that combines water with natural ingredients is going to provide good food for bacteria, and so preservatives are a must in shampoos. The most common ones in shampoos are parabens. Another common preservative is the tongue-twisting methyl chloroisothiazolinone.

Chelating agents. The letters EDTA on a shampoo label indicate that the product contains a chelating agent. These are ingredients that attract and hold minerals from water and other ingredients in the product, enhancing the product's foaming ability and preventing the minerals from depositing on the hair and leaving a dull finish.

Vitamins. Often manufacturers add vitamins to shampoos, claiming that they can help to "nourish the hair from within." Experts are mixed on whether or not vitamins in shampoos can really help hair. Some doctors point out that hair is dead and therefore can't be "nourished." Others note that most vitamins are too large to penetrate the hair shaft and have any effect on the hair. Some cosmetic chemists point out, however, that vitamin E in shampoo and conditioners can have antioxidizing effects on the hair, helping to protect color-treated hair from discoloration due to sun exposure, chlorinated water, or other environmental hazards. Panthenol (vitamin B-5) is thought to be able to penetrate the hair shaft and strengthen the hair.

Sunscreens. Because they are washed out before one goes into the sun, sunscreens (such as benzophenones, salicylates, and cinnamates) are not thought to be very helpful in shampoos. In products such as leave-in conditioners they may be of greater benefit, particularly for color-treated or permed hair, which can become sun-damaged more easily than "virgin" hair.

Balsam. This fragrant resinous substance oozes naturally from many different plants and can add body and volume to the hair, particularly when combined with proteins.

Herbs. In many instances herbs are included just to add fragrance to a product, or to make it sound more "natural" and appealing. But when used in high enough concentrations, certain herbs can have direct effects on hair. Camomile, a yellow extract, can brighten the hair slightly. Capsicum extract and juniper extract can have an invigorating effect on the scalp. Rosemary is thought to help cut oiliness in the hair and scalp.

Citric acid. Sometimes added to neutralize the alkaline pH, citric acid makes a shampoo more appropriate for use on color-treated, permed, or straightened hair. By smoothing out the cuticle of hair, citric acid also makes hair appear shinier.

Honey. Because its high sugar concentration draws and holds onto water, honey is a natural moisturizer. Some experts note, however, that the effects of honey in a shampoo are washed away in the rinse, leaving no lasting benefits on the hair. Still, it has a marketing advantage, making the product sound more natural and "healthy."

Colors and fragrances. These are usually listed very obviously on the label, just as "fragrance" or, in the case of colors, with dye names such as "FD&C Yellow No. 5." They add only to the esthetic appeal of the product, not to the product's efficacy. Still, some manufacturers believe that the scent of a shampoo can be its key selling point.

Now that you've got the basics of what's in a shampoo, how do you choose one? If you're like many women, your hair fits many of the categories that separate one shampoo from another. Your hair may be color-treated *and* fine and limp, *and* you may wash it every day. So do you choose a shampoo for color-treated hair? Or one that builds body? Or one that is created just for daily washing?

David Cannell, Ph.D., vice president of technology at Redken Laboratories, says you should go in the order of what is your hair's biggest problem. "You should consider damage first, then diameter, then lifestyle," says Dr. Cannell. "So in this case you should choose a shampoo and conditioner for color-treated hair; once you treat the damage, the other problems will seem less important."

Whether you choose to buy your shampoo at your hair

salon or the drugstore probably won't make much difference in terms of the product itself; there are fine shampoos available at both places. Your hairstylist, because of his or her familiarity with your hair, may be able to suggest shampoos that can work well with your hair type and style. Salon products do tend to be more expensive, however, and if you have had success using a drugstore-brand product, you're probably just as well off continuing to use it.

Shampoos for Different Hair Types

What are the real differences among shampoos marketed toward specific hair types? Again, the answer lies in the way the products are balanced.

Shampoos for color-treated hair and/or permed or chemically straightened hair. Generally, these processes use alkaline solutions to cause permanent changes in the hair and, in so doing, open up the hair cuticle, making it more porous, brittle, and dry. Shampoos for this type of hair, then, will have a low alkalinity (and a low pH factor, under 7) to keep the hair firm and compact. They may also be rich in conditioners, but not so rich that they weigh down the hair (particularly for permed hair).

Body-building shampoos. Often these are formulated to remove the buildup of styling products, which can weigh down your hair and make it appear limp and lifeless. These shampoos may therefore have a higher level of surfactants and fewer oils and moisturizing ingredients. They may also have proteins and polymers designed to coat the hair and add thickness and body.

Moisturizing shampoos. Designed for dry, brittle hair, moisturizing shampoos may contain a high level of humectants, such as sugars and amino acids or glycerin. They also have a lower level of surfactants in order to prevent excessive stripping of the hair's natural oils.

Therapeutic shampoos. Shampoos designed to treat certain scalp or hair conditions usually contain one "active" ingredient in addition to the basic substances the shampoo comprises. There are six ingredients that are FDA-approved for treating dandruff and/or psoriasis or seborrhea. They include zinc pyrithione, sulfur, selenium sulfide, coal tar extract, salicylic acid, and the combination of sulfur and salicylic acid. (For more information on these conditions and ingredients, see Chapter 9, pages 148–149.)

Daily wash shampoos. Because they are formulated to be lower in detergents and higher in moisturizing ingredients, daily wash shampoos may not clean the hair thoroughly enough for women who use many styling products, but they are effective for light cleansing.

Shampoo-and-conditioner-in-one products. Shampoos with conditioner built in are formulated primarily for women whose hair is in fairly good shape and who want to be able to cut down the amount of time they need to spend in the shower. These products have surfactants for cleansing the hair plus special silicones that are designed to stay on the hair even through rinsing; the silicones act as conditioning agents, coating the hair shaft and making it easier to comb. Most experts agree that these shampoos compromise somewhat on quality while maximizing convenience; the cleansing action won't be as good as that of a regular shampoo, and the conditioning won't be as thorough as that of a regular conditioner. But in a pinch, these products can provide adequate cleansing and conditioning.

What about shampoos that promise to "self-adjust," providing conditioning where you need it and cleansing where you need it? In fact, no shampoo can really do that. If anything, the hair adjusts to the shampoo; the more porous parts of the hair may naturally absorb conditioners and other ingredients more readily than the healthier hair at the roots. (For more on this, see the next section.)

Getting the Most from Your Shampoo

Studies show that most women have two or three shampoos in their bathrooms at any one time. This makes sense because it is a good idea to switch shampoos every few days. If you usually use a moisturizing shampoo, switch to a more thorough cleansing shampoo every few days to clear away the product buildup that your usual shampoo can't break down. Or if your hair is becoming dry from your usual cleansing shampoo, switch to a moisturizing shampoo every few days to add softness back into your hair.

Since most women shampoo more frequently (even once or twice a day) than they used to, the old advice of "lathering twice" is no longer necessary, and many shampoo companies have taken it off their labels; since there's less buildup of dirt and oils, most shampoos will do a thorough cleansing job with just one lathering and rinsing. It's best to get your hair uniformly wet first, then massage just a small amount of shampoo throughout your hair, letting it blend with the water and form a rich lather. Rinse hair thoroughly with warm water, waiting until the water runs clear into the drain. The harder your water is (and the more minerals it contains), the longer rinsing is likely to take. But thorough rinsing is key to thorough cleansing and to preventing a dull finish on the hair.

Conditioners: Deep vs. Daily

Many women over thirty can remember the days before the word *conditioner* came into being, and we used "cream rinses" to detangle our hair. Today's daily or instant conditioners serve essentially the same purpose as those early cream rinses, but they contain high-tech ingredients that weren't used in those simple rinses. As a result, they can achieve effects in the hair—ranging from building body to protecting color—that simple cream rinses could not.

Like shampoos, conditioners have to perform a balancing act. They have to leave behind enough ingredients so that the hair combs easily and feels soft and touchable but not so much that the hair looks weighed down, limp, or, heaven forbid, "greasy."

How does a conditioner work? Basically, all conditioners are positively charged and, as such, are drawn to the negative charges of the surface of the hair. The more damaged a woman's hair is, the stronger the negative charge of her hair and the greater the attraction to the conditioner. Once the conditioner has "stuck" to the hair, particularly to the more dried-out parts, it provides slip and reduces the friction of the hair, making it easier to comb.

Most conditioners either have an oil base or are oil-free with a polymer base. A typical polymer ingredient might be something like polyquaternium 10; often the oil base is a chloride ingredient, for example, trimethyl cetyl ammonium chloride. Today most conditioners also contain silicones, which can add shine to the hair.

Conditioners that promise to "build body" are likely to have a lot of proteins, which stick to the hair, adding bulk without oil. Moisturizing conditioners (which may also be the conditioners for dry, damaged, or color-treated hair) are likely to contain amino acids, sugars, small proteins, and other ingredients that can draw and hold moisture to the hair.

All cream conditioners also contain emulsifiers (such as glyceryl stearate or cetyl alcohol) and the same preservatives and fragrances that you're likely to find in shampoos.

The big difference between a deep conditioner and a daily conditioner (or what some manufacturers call a hair "treatment," and a hair "rinse") is that deep conditioners tend to have more concentrated ingredients and the ingredients tend to be of smaller molecular weight, which allows the deep conditioner to penetrate more easily into the hair shaft during the twenty minutes or so you leave it on. Daily conditioners are meant to be washed away with every shampoo and therefore don't need to penetrate into the hair shaft; instead, they coat the hair with detangling ingredients.

Making the Most of Your Conditioner

If you use a conditioner according to directions and your hair still appears limp and oily, you may have chosen the wrong type of conditioner for your hair, or you may be applying too much, or you may not be rinsing thoroughly.

Before switching to another type of conditioner, try going one day without it (to eliminate any buildup that might have occurred on your hair) and then apply conditioner only to the parts of your hair that really need it—usually the dry, split ends that tangle easily and can make hair appear fly-away—rather than throughout your hair. Rinse the conditioner until the water runs clear. If this doesn't work, try a different kind of conditioner, one designed to build body rather than to moisturize hair, and again be careful not to apply too much.

If, on the other hand, your hair seems dry and brittle even after you have used a daily conditioner, try using a deep conditioner. If this seems to make your hair softer and more manageable, plan to use it once a week or so until your hair gets back into good shape.

Deep conditioners can also help you to get the most out of a perm or coloring process. If you deep-condition your hair once a week for two or three weeks before you have the processing done, your hair will have fewer porous spots, and the perm or color will go on more evenly, with less chance of overprocessing, and less additional damage due to the processing.

Some stylists also recommend combing a daily or deep conditioner throughout your wet hair and leaving it in if you're planning to spend a day at the beach. The conditioner will help to prevent damage from sun, salt, and chlorine and will keep your hair looking neat while you are there. And the heat of the sun will help the conditioner to penetrate the hair, so that you'll be giving your hair a treatment while you relax.

The New Styling Tools—Mousses, Gels, and More

The days of sleeping with rollers in our hair and baking our heads under beehive-shaped dryers are (thank heaven) over for most of us. In place of the structured hairstyles of decades ago have come softer, easier looks and with them a whole new "generation" of styling products—mousses, gels, lotions, spritzes, and hairsprays.

Basically all styling products have the same purpose: to form a film on the hair that will hold the hair in the shape of a certain desired style. In order to do this, all styling products have a polymer base—that is, a base of materials that are made of large molecules all strung together. Our ancestors held their hair in place with gelatins and starch—natural polymers. The molecules in today's polymer bases in styling products may be proteins, starchlike ingredients, silicones, or totally synthetic substances.

The polymer is put in a solution of water or alcohol. Products that promise "firm hold" or "extra hold" are almost always in an alcohol base because these types of polymers are soluble only in alcohol. Alcohol may also be the secret to styling products that help hair to dry faster. Some manufacturers boast of "no alcohol" styling products, claiming that alcohol dries out the hair because as it evaporates, it takes water with it. But some cosmetic chemists note that hair quickly adjusts to the ambient humidity and reabsorbs the water, so that alcohol really isn't a great consideration in choosing a styling product.

Water-soluble products tend to be the lighter-weight, lighter-hold products. They may work well for uncomplicated styles or just for combing hair in place, but they won't offer the staying power of alcohol-based styling lotions.

Mousses, in addition to their polymer base, also contain surfactants, detergent materials that produce the foamlike mousse. Today cosmetic technology has led to the development of silicone plasticizers and different surfactants that can be combined in different ways to make a product have stronger hold or more elasticity, so that hair can be easily brushed even after the mousse or gel or spritz has been applied.

In general, mousses or light gels offer the lightest hold (although, again, the alcohol-based varieties tend to be stronger), styling lotions are next in line, firm gels are next, and then spritzes and hairsprays tend to offer the greatest hold.

All of these products offer some styling benefits to the hair and may even protect the hair from excessive heat due to blow dryers, curling irons, and hot rollers. (Some even contain silicone ingredients specifically designed to dissipate heat throughout the hair, preventing too much from hitting any one area.) Which product you choose to use will depend on your hair type, the style you want to achieve, and the degree of hold you need. Some women use only hairspray, applied once their hair is dried and in place. Other women prefer the flexibility of a mousse or styling lotion, which may not provide as firm a hold as hairspray but will keep the hair more "touchable."

Whatever you choose, the key is not to use too much and not to have too many different products on your hair at once, which can cause product buildup. You'll know if there is a buildup of products on your hair because it will feel sticky or greasy and will look weighed down and dull. If you do have product buildup, try switching to a more cleansing shampoo than you usually use.

Brushing Up

Despite what Grandma told you, the old advice of brushing your hair one hundred times a night to add shine may actually do more harm to the hair than good. While regular brushing can help to distribute natural oils throughout the hair (adding shine) and may add body temporarily to your hair (particularly if you brush while bending over, from the back of your neck to the ends of your hair), brushing too frequently or for too long may increase your risks of damaging your hair, particularly if you use a brush with sharp, pointy bristles, which can cut into the hair and cause breakage.

What is important is choosing the right brush and comb for your hair and styling needs, using them carefully and gently, and keeping them clean and maintained. Most stylists agree on the following points:

- Choose a brush with round-ended bristles—whether they're natural or plastic. Replace the brush as soon as most of the rounded tips have broken off.

- Opt for a wide-toothed comb, no matter what type of hair you have. It will detangle your hair with a minimum of breakage.

- If your cut requires a lot of styling with a brush, choose one with a rubber or vinyl handle (they're slip-proof).

- If you use your brush while blow-drying your hair, choose a brush with vents; they allow warm air to circulate to your hair, cutting down on drying time.

- Never use a brush to detangle wet hair; this could cause extensive damage to the hair. Instead, use a wide-toothed comb, and comb the hair in small sections, starting at the bottom of the hair and working your way up to the scalp.

- Keep your brush and comb clean by pulling out hairs every time you use them and giving them a once-a-week soak in warm water and a few drops of ammonia.

- Never share your brush or comb with anyone else. Some organisms, not to mention oils and debris, can easily be transmitted from their hair to yours or vice versa.

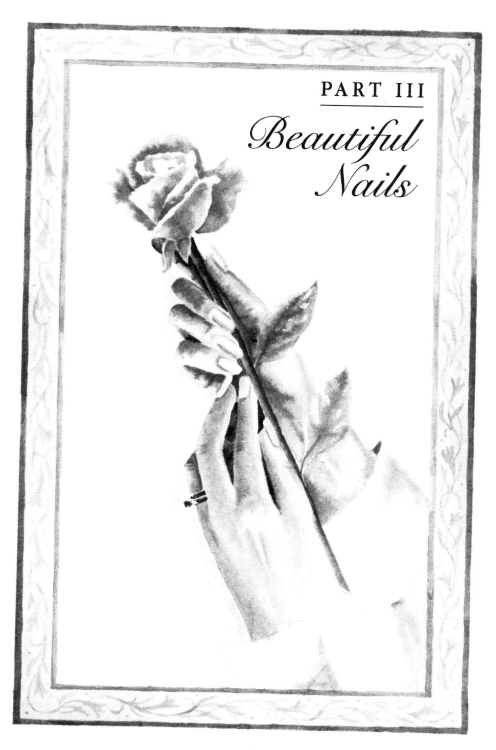

PART III
Beautiful Nails

CHAPTER 11

The Five Ages of Your Nails

If, as Scarlett O'Hara's mother warned, "You can always tell a lady by her hands," then well-groomed nails could be the finishing touch to a flawless image. Throughout your life your nails will be one reflection of your well-being—both mental and physical. Personnel recruiters often note that they look at a prospective employee's fingernails for clues to how well the person manages stress and how carefully she attends to detail. (Bitten, manipulated-looking nails often indicate someone who is nervous, overstressed, and less attentive to her appearance than she should be.) And men and women in general often look at each other's hands for clues to just how well one takes care of oneself.

The Anatomy of Nails

Nails are made up of the same proteinous substance—keratin—that is in your skin and hair. This protein contains sulfur, the element that makes nails hard and rigid. Like hair, nails are composed of dead cells, which means that they don't hurt when you cut them and also that they can't be "nourished" by anything that is applied to them to make them grow faster, longer, stronger, or thicker. Nails protect our fingers and toes from injury, aid our manual dexterity, and are helpful when we have an itch. Like skin and hair, nails can regenerate if they are injured or cut, and they can reflect inner health—or sickness.

Nails are composed of five parts. The nail plate is what

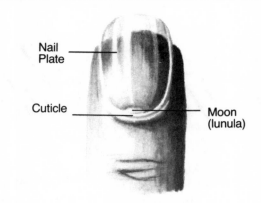

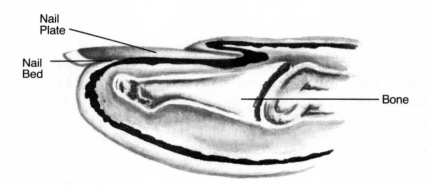

you think of when you consider nails; it's what you file. Right underneath the nail plate is the nail bed—a soft bed of skin that contains the blood vessels that nourish the nail plate and give it its pinkish color. At the bottom of the nail plate is the cuticle, a fold of skin that seals the nail to the skin, preventing dirt, bacteria and other substances from getting into the nail and its growth center, the matrix, which is located directly under the cuticle. The matrix is the area under the cuticle where cells of the nail plate are regenerated. Keeping the matrix intact is critical to the healthy growth of your nails. The white "half moon" at the base of each of your nails is known as the lunula, but it is actually the visible part of the matrix. Below the nail bed is the bone of the finger and the fat layer of skin.

Fingernails grow an average of one-eighth to one-quarter

inch per month, and complete nail turnover takes three to six months. (Toenails require two to three times longer to grow from base to tip.) Nails also grow faster during warm weather than during cold, and they grow faster in typists and pianists than in the general population. They also grow faster in children than in adults, and in men than in women. This fast growth could be the result of increased circulation to the fingertips, but no one knows for certain. Interestingly, the longer your fingers are, the faster your nails grow; the nails on the middle fingers tend to grow most quickly, while thumb and "pinkie" nails tend to grow most slowly. Nails also grow more quickly on your "dominant" hand, that is, your right hand if you're right-handed. Some women believe that high stress slows nail growth, but there is no scientific evidence to support this belief.

The Five Ages of Your Nails

The rate of nail growth and the health of nails vary at different times of one's life. Just as we can see changes in a woman's skin as she ages, so can we see changes in her nails. And just as certain habits such as sunbathing can exacerbate natural aging of the skin, so can they accelerate aging in nails. The following is a typical lifeline of toenails and fingernails.

Infancy

Nails begin to grow at about twelve weeks of fetal development in the womb. By the time a baby is born, her nails are fully formed and are softer and more flexible than at any other time in her life. They also grow rapidly and must be clipped regularly, probably once or twice a week, to keep the baby from scratching herself. Blunt scissors, baby nail clippers, or even a soft emery board should do the trick. Keep fingernails rounded at the sides; toenails should be cut straight across. If your baby is very active, it may be best to clip her nails when she is sleeping so that you don't accidentally catch you or your baby with the scissors.

Often a newborn's toenails look ingrown because the skin around them is puffy and soft. If the skin around a toenail looks inflamed and the baby seems to experience pain when you touch the area, consult your pediatrician. (Always call your physician if the toe itself becomes swollen; in rare cases a hair can get wound around the toe, almost imperceptibly, and if left to tighten long enough, it can cut off circulation to the toe. Removing the hair requires medical attention.) Usually ingrown toenails resolve by themselves; sometimes applying warm compresses may help guide the nail out over the skin, but it's best to seek medical attention before doing anything more drastic. Because toenails grow more slowly than fingernails (at all stages of life), they don't need to be trimmed as frequently as fingernails.

Childhood

Considering all the unappealing things that small kids get into—from sandboxes and mud pies to bugs and animals of all sorts—it's a pleasant surprise that nail problems in small children are relatively uncommon. Some doctors chalk that up to the fact that kids' nails grow rapidly and don't give fungus and bacteria a chance to start up a colony as easily as they do in slower-growing nails.

One of the most common problems that occurs in children, usually beginning about age five or six, is nail-biting. Doctors are unsure just how common nail-biting is, but it's generally thought to be related to stress. Not only does nail-biting look unattractive, but it can lead to increased risks of inflammation and infection of the nail and the skin around it. Stopping the habit isn't always easy. There are some nail-polish-like products on the market that, when applied to the nails, give them a bitter, unpleasant taste. Dermatologists don't have any evidence that these actually work, but they may be worth a try.

Parents can often discourage nail-biting in young girls by supplying them with attractive manicuring utensils and teaching them how to groom and care for their nails properly. Some doctors recommend trying to find and eliminate the source of the stress that's causing the child to bite her nails in the first place. On the bright side, nails grow faster in nail-biters, although no one knows exactly why. It's possible that the healing process that follows any trauma to the nails just naturally speeds up the growth rate. Most people stop nail-biting by the time they reach adulthood.

Injuries to the nails are fairly common in childhood. Often they result in white spots on the nail plate or black or blue color underneath the nail. The darker colors indicate that bleeding has occurred under the nail, and it should be looked at by a physician, especially if the child is experiencing pain.

Children who suck their thumbs sometimes get yeast infections in the nails, a condition known by the medical name candida paronychia. (Candida is the name of the invading organism, and paronychia is the medical term for inflammation of the nail folds.) The constant moisture on the thumb and nail makes a perfect environment for yeast to thrive. The condition can usually be treated with a local antifungal medication, but most doctors also recommend trying to break the child of the thumb-sucking habit.

Although it's uncommon, some children may develop a mole underneath a nail, which usually appears as a long band of pigment within the nail plate. If the mole looks very dark or black, the doctor may want to biopsy it to eliminate the possibility of melanoma.

In children with psoriasis, the nail surface may appear cracked or pitted, and the nail plate may separate from the nail bed. Again, such symptoms should be brought to your dermatologist's attention.

Adolescence

Nails appear to be much less affected by the changing hormones in adolescence than skin and hair. There's no significant change in nail growth patterns or in nail health in most teenagers. However, unusual teenage habits can be reflected in nails. For example, a teenage girl who experiments with crash diets or who experiences an eating disorder may have very brittle nails that crack and break easily. In fact, such symptoms in nails may be one tip-off that a teenage girl has anorexia (a condition in which she will deny herself food in an effort to take control of her body). The brittleness is due to extreme dietary deficiencies caused by inadequate diet.

In people who eat a well-balanced diet, dietary changes don't have any noticeable effect, with one possible exception; recent studies have shown that supplementation with the nutrient biotin, found naturally in such foods as egg yolk, dark-green vegetables, and liver, may help make fingernails less brittle. Biotin is known to be important to healthy hair, skin, and nails. There is not yet enough evidence about biotin, however, to suggest universal supplementation for everyone. If you have problems with very brittle nails, discuss the possibility of taking biotin supplements with your doctor. Just for the record, there is no evidence that consuming gelatin will strengthen, harden, or make nails grow in healthier or faster.

The teenage years are also often the first time that problems associated with overmanipulative manicures begin. Cutting back the cuticles too far and performing manicures too frequently can cause nail infections, dryness, and trauma to the nail. (For more information, see Chapter 3.) Often it's best to allow a teenage girl to have one professional manicure to learn the correct way to take care of her nails.

Teenagers experience more ingrown toenails than any other age group. The reason probably has to do with the fact that increased physical activity and sweating cause the skin around the toes to become puffy and swollen, making the nail more likely to push into the skin. (For advice on how to treat an ingrown toenail, see Chapter 13, pages 188–189.)

Twenties to Forties: The Reproductive Years

During the thirty years from your early twenties to the end of your forties, the growth rate of your nails will most likely slow down. Nails may also appear a bit thicker and even less smooth, sometimes forming ridges along the nail plate. These are normal changes associated with a general slowing down of your body's metabolism.

You may also notice that your nails grow faster premenstrually and during menstruation and that they seem to grow fastest during pregnancy, especially the early months of pregnancy. Doctors don't know exactly why this is so. There's been some speculation that increased estrogen during these times can stimulate nail growth, but no one knows for certain. Nail growth tends to slow down again sometime in the months following pregnancy.

Fifty-Plus

After menopause, changes in nails seem to become slightly more obvious. Nail growth rate continues to slow, and nails become thicker. Often nails will form ridges. "I believe that the ridges in nails in an older person are analogous to the wrinkles in skin as a sign of aging," says Richard K. Scher, M.D., professor of dermatology and head of the nail section at Columbia Presbyterian Medical Center. "And there's some evidence that excessive sun exposure can cause damage to the elastic tissue of the nail bed, just as it can to the skin; in my experience the women who have the most facial wrinkles also tend to have the most nail ridges, and they've usually spent a lot of time in the sun."

A lifetime of smoking can also take its toll by the time you enter your fifties. Nails may become permanently yellowed, stained by the tars in cigarettes. Some doctors also believe that the negative effects of cigarette smoking on circulation can slow nail growth rate even more than natural aging can; the less blood you have flowing to your fingernails, the more slowly they're going to grow.

Nails may also become more brittle and more likely to crack as you age, a fact that doctors attribute to a decreased water content in the nail. The slower rate of turnover of the nails also means that they may be thicker; you may need to soak your fingers and toes in warm water for fifteen or twenty minutes in order to soften the nails so that they can be cut more easily.

Fungal infections of fingernails and especially of toenails also become much more common as one ages. The increase may be due in part to the slowed-down growth rate of the nails, which gives the fungi more time to grow, but some doctors feel that increased infections reflect the fact that the immune system in general is just less effective as we age. Keeping nails cut short, clean, and dry should help to prevent fungal infections. And using an antifungal powder in shoes can help too.

Some women claim that their nails grow faster and look better after they begin estrogen replacement therapy. To date, however, there is no good evidence that this is true.

CHAPTER 12

Nail Problems and Overall Health

If, as the saying goes, the eyes are the windows to the soul, then nails may be the portholes to the inside of the body. Today a skilled dermatologist can look at your fingernails and toenails for clues to whether or not you've experienced disorders ranging from heart attack or lung cancer to anemia or pneumonia. For this reason many health experts today advocate a thorough examination of the nails during regular checkups and during dermatological checkups. In addition, you should be aware of signs of trouble in your own nails. The vast majority of symptoms are nothing to worry about; usually they result from minor trauma to the nail and disappear when the nail has completely grown out (in about six months). Symptoms may be unsightly or, in occasional cases, may signal an underlying physical problem. Any persistent symptoms should always be brought to your physician's attention. Here are some common problems and what they mean.

Brittle Nails

Some dermatologists who specialize in nail care claim that this is the most common problem that women bring to their offices. Women with very brittle nails may notice that their nails will split lengthwise down the nail or the nail will split off in shinglelike pieces. Nail brittleness is analogous to dry skin and often occurs at the same time; it's more common in women with dry skin than in those with oily skin. The problem is basically an inability of the nails to hold water. One reason is that, unlike skin and hair, nails contain very little fat and oils to hold in moisture. Brittle nails tend to worsen in the wintertime, when cold dry air and dehydrating indoor heat can add to the ambient dryness and pull more water out of the skin, hair, and nails. Although wearing nail polish is one way to minimize water evaporation from the nails, helping to prevent brittleness, too-frequent manicures (more than once a week) may increase risks of brittleness; nail polish removers contain solvents that can strip nails of their natural moisture, making them drier and brittleness more likely.

The answer to brittle nails is to add water and oils to the nails. Soak your nails once or twice a day in warm (not hot!) water; you should be able to feel your nails soften, an indication that they are absorbing some of the water. Immediately follow the soak with an application of a rich hand cream, preferably one that contains phospholipids or ingredients such as urea or lactic acid. At night wear soft cotton gloves to bed on occasion to help keep the moisturizer on your hands, not on your bed linens. Since household detergents can strip natural oils from hands and nails, be sure to wear cotton-lined vinyl gloves whenever you do any housework that involves cleaning chemicals.

Researchers are also conducting ongoing studies of different substances that may help to make nails less brittle. One is the supplement biotin, as discussed earlier. In one study conducted by Swiss dermatologists, patients with brittle nails who took supplements of biotin experienced stronger, thicker, smoother nails within nine months.

In the United States, researchers at Columbia Presbyterian Medical Center in New York have been studying the use of the hair growth drug minoxidil in nails. The studies were spurred by anecdotal reports that people who rubbed minoxidil into their scalps with their fingertips experienced less brittle, more durable nails. Preliminary research hasn't been very encouraging, but the doctors are continuing to look into the possible connection between minoxidil and less brittle nails.

In rare cases brittle nails can be one sign of internal conditions such as poor circulation, arthritis, or dietary deficiency. For this reason alert your doctor to any persistent unusual brittleness of your nails.

Nail Clubbing

Nail clubbing is a defect that changes the normal angle of the nail and the way the nail sits on the nail bed. If you look at your fingernails from the perspective of the side of your finger, you'll see that your nail plate angles slightly downward into the cuticle area of your finger. In clubbed nails, the nail plate slants upward into the cuticle area. In addition, in normal nails, if you press down on the nail, the nail will feel hard and solid. In clubbed nails, when pressing down on the nail plate, you'd feel a sponginess or springiness to the nail bed.

What do these changes mean? Diseases of the heart and lung may lead to nail clubbing, and very painful clubbing that begins suddenly and abruptly may in rare cases be one sign of cancer, particularly lung cancer. For these reasons nail clubbing should always be checked by your doctor.

Spoon Fingernails

Nails that develop spoonlike depressions in their centers may be subtle signs that a woman is anemic or is experiencing a thyroid imbalance, and they warrant a checkup with your physician, particularly if they occur in several nails at a time.

Hangnails

Hangnails are not really part of the nail at all but are small pieces of the skin around the nail that have been cut or torn and can protrude. They can get caught on things like nail files or your hosiery and often feel quite tender and painful. Most people feel they are unattractive and should be removed. What's the proper way to remove them? *Not* by pulling or biting the skin away. These methods only raise your risk of infection. Instead, gently clip the hangnail with manicure scissors or cuticle clippers, and if the area seems inflamed, apply a small amount of bacterial ointment.

Minimize your chances of hangnails in the future by

- Being careful when doing manicures not to overcut the cuticles.

- Keeping nails and hands well moisturized whenever possible; hangnails are more likely to occur in dry skin.

- Not using your fingernails as tools; make it a habit to use letter openers and other helpful tools to prevent paper cuts and other injury to the nail area.

Nail Ridges

We've already discussed the fact that ridges that run lengthwise on your nails can be a sign of aging, akin to wrinkles in the skin. Heredity is thought to play a role in your likelihood of developing these ridges, just as it plays a role in how much you will wrinkle. Many women begin to notice ridges in their fingernails once they pass age thirty, but the ridges often grow more prominent with age.

Lengthwise ridges can also result from overzealous manicures or injury to the nail, which can cause damage to the matrix of the nail or the nail bed, resulting in temporary deformation of the nail plate in the form of ridges. Again, careful manicuring should prevent most nail ridge problems. When in doubt, do too little to nails, not too much.

Sometimes injury to the cuticle area produces horizontal furrows known as Beau's lines, which follow the lunula shape of the nail. If the Beau's lines appear in all of the nails at once, however, they are likely to be due to an internal problem, not an injury to the nail. The horizontal lines can result from severe sickness, malnutrition, chemotherapy, or carpal tunnel syndrome (a neurologic disorder that affects the hands and fingers).

Nail ridges can also be due to eczema or psoriasis of the hand and on occasion may appear after a serious illness, such as pneumonia, which can temporarily halt nail growth. Very obvious ridges that seem to arise fairly suddenly and involve several fingernails should be looked at by your dermatologist.

Slow-Growing Nails

As mentioned in Chapter 11, nails grow at different rates throughout our lives—faster during warm weather and during pregnancy and slowing down postpartum, in cold weather, and with age. A sudden reduction in the rate of nail growth, however, could signal trouble. Nail growth slows dramatically during times of high fever, for example, or after a heart attack or any other severe traumatic event (including, as mentioned, the birth of a baby). Contrary to some cosmetic claims, there's nothing you can apply that will speed up the rate of nail growth. Keeping nails well manicured and protecting them from mechanical damage will help to keep them looking good. Slow-growing nails are not considered a serious medical concern, but as a reflection of your inner health, they should be monitored and discussed with your physician.

Yellow or Brown Nails

Yellow or brownish tints on your nails are rarely cause for concern. They are most often due to the use of deeply pigmented nail enamels. Use of polish remover probably won't get rid of the stain because the pigment can get embedded into the nail plate, leaving the shadow of the original tint of the polish. The color will fade naturally over a few weeks if you leave nails bare during this time. To speed up the process, try buffing the tops of the nails very gently with a soft nail buffer or with the soft side of your emery board. The buffing works like exfoliation on the skin, removing the topmost cell layers of the nail and exposing fresher layers below. Some manicurists also recommend applying lemon juice to bleach the yellow color out of the nail.

Sometimes whitening agents can be applied just under nail tips to give the illusion of whiter nails. Nail yellowing from dark polishes can often be avoided in the future by applying one or two clear base coats under the colored polish to act as a shield between the pigment and your nail.

Nails and fingers can also become yellow from contact with certain substances, such as tars from cigarettes, hair dyes, and even wet rusty metal. Long-term use of the antibiotic tetracycline can also produce nails that are yellow and thick. Again, the yellowing should fade naturally if you avoid these substances for a few weeks.

Nail yellowing that persists despite your best efforts for removal may signal respiratory illness or lung or kidney disorders in rare cases. See your physician.

White or Dark Spots on Nails

Nail injuries are fairly common, and considering how much we all use our fingers, it's surprising that they aren't more so. Two of the most frequent problems that result from injuries to nails are white or black spots on the nail. If the injury has caused bleeding under the nail, the spot is likely to be black or deep blue in color. It's a sign that the bleeding has stopped and a scab has formed. Such scabs may cause part of the nail around the injury to loosen from the nail bed, opening the door to further infection. To minimize problems from this separation of the nail bed, leave the nail alone and prevent it from coming into contact with any irritating substances, such as household cleaning agents or detergents.

Keep the nails dry during the day and apply petroleum jelly in the evening to soothe and protect the area. Do not polish the nail or cover it with a fake fingernail.

Blue skin that appears below the lunula area at the base of the nail may signal poor circulation, heart disease, or lung disease and should be brought to your physician's attention. In rare cases malignant melanoma can also strike the fingers and the nails. It will appear as brown or black discoloration under the nail, sometimes extending to the surrounding fingers. Such symptoms warrant immediate medical attention.

Women with dark complexions are more likely than fair-skinned individuals to develop dark lines in their nails that run lengthwise. The lines are caused by the deposit of pigment by the skin's pigment cells, the melanocytes. Although no one knows just what causes these lines to occur, they are only rarely considered to be a medical problem.

White spots in nails can also be due to injury and often signal that the nail has separated from the nail bed. If the spots appear on only one or two nails, they are probably the result of trauma to the nail and will simply grow out as the nail replaces itself. If the spots appear on all of the nails and also on the toenails, they may signal a dietary deficiency of calcium and/or zinc or a medical condition such as psoriasis. See your physician.

Splinter Hemorrhages

Red streaks that run lengthwise along the nail may be splinter hemorrhages caused by trauma to the nail or by something more serious. When they occur at the nail tip and affect only one or two nails, they are most likely caused by trauma. When they affect many or all of the nails at once and occur closer to the cuticle, they can suggest an internal disease such as vasculitis (inflamation of blood vessels) or endocarditis (a disorder of a heart valve). Consult a doctor if you have these latter symptoms.

Fungal Infections

Toenails and fingernails that appear thickened, ridged, yellow, and dull may be infected with fungi or bacteria. These infections are especially likely to occur following breakage to the skin around the nail, which can allow bacteria to get into the nail, or in people whose feet or hands are frequently wet, creating an environment where these organisms can thrive. Fungal infections are most common in older adults but can occur at any time in one's life. Your doctor may prescribe an antifungal cream and/or oral antibiotics to treat the problem. Most infections clear up with use of these products. Wearing socks that are designed to wick moisture away from the skin also helps to minimize fungal infections, as does wearing shoes that are not too tight.

Ingrown Toenails

Like so many nail problems, ingrown toenails result most often from our efforts to make our feet look better—by cutting toenails too short or shaping them improperly and by wearing narrow, pinching shoes that press in on our toes. Cutting toenails too short or in a curved fashion can cause the sharp edges of the toenail to press into the skin around it as it grows out. Tight shoes exacerbate the problem by pressing that skin further into the nail. Most common in the big toes, ingrown toenails can become so tender that even the slightest touch can cause shooting pain. In the worst cases they can become severely infected, oozing pus and causing severe swelling.

Prevention of ingrown toenails begins with proper pedicures (see Chapter 13, page 193, for details) and with properly fitting shoes. Try on shoes at the end of the day, to allow room for the natural swelling that occurs in feet throughout the day. Look for shoes with wide, rounded toeboxes and avoid heel heights of more than one or at most two inches.

The higher your heels, the more you're pushing your toes into a smaller area. (High heels can also cause back pain and damage the muscles and tendons in the foot and legs; avoid them.) When doing any extended walking or exercising, choose a roomy, sneakerlike sport shoe with good support and cushioning.

Sometimes you can treat minor ingrown toenails yourself. Soak your feet for fifteen minutes or so in warm water mixed with Epsom salts to soften the skin around the nail. Then gently push the skin away from the nail with a soft cloth or your fingertip. (Do not insert any sharp instrument into the area to push the skin aside.) Apply a small amount of sterile cotton underneath the nail or between the nail and the skin to help the nail grow out and away from the skin and to help the surrounding skin heal. Do this twice a day if possible until the nail grows out and the skin heals completely.

If the infection is very painful, persistent, or if you notice a puslike discharge, see your physician. Also see your physician if you are diabetic and have any toenail disorder. Some diabetics develop nerve disorders that decrease the sensitivity of their feet, so that even a serious advanced infection can cause no pain and therefore runs the risk of going unattended. Left unattended, the ingrown toenail can lead to severe infection.

Nails and AIDS

People who have AIDS (autoimmune deficiency syndrome) often experience changes in their nails as well as in their hair and skin. Such changes may include severe or unusual fungal infections that involve all of the fingers at once or both palms; nail thickening and/or ridging and loosening of the nails from the nail beds; whitening of the nails or, if the person is taking the drug AZT, blue nails. Persistent wartlike lesions and squamous cell cancers of the fingers are also possible. These symptoms are rarely the only signs that one has AIDS, but they certainly merit medical attention.

CHAPTER 13

A Perfect Ten: Manicure Guidelines

If left alone, fingernails and toenails in most healthy women look and feel just fine. Most nail problems are self-inflicted. The biggest offender? Poorly performed manicures. In an effort to make our nails look neater, shinier, or flashier, we all too often can make them look worse by such mistakes as cutting back cuticles too far and trimming them unevenly. Here are the proper ways to do a manicure and a pedicure, along with vital tips on what to look for in a nail salon to make sure it's the best place you can go for professional nail care.

First, some general safety tips. Manicures should be done no more frequently than once a week. Too-frequent application and removal of nail products can make nails dry and brittle and raise the risk for irritation of the skin around the nails. Don't share manicure utensils or products with others unless they have been sterilized between uses; you could spread infection. If you have little ones around the house, keep all manicuring products out of reach. Nail polish enamel and remover can be toxic if ingested, and some of the utensils—files, cuticle clippers, orange sticks—can cause injuries easily.

Your Nail Care Tool Kit

The best start to a good manicure or pedicure is having the right utensils and keeping them in top shape. Here are guidelines to stocking your nail care arsenal.

Nail clippers or scissors may be used for trimming nails. Most experts recommend nail clippers for toenails, scissors for fingernails if you don't want to file them. Keep both clean by wiping them with cotton soaked in rubbing alcohol after each use and storing them in a closed, dust-proof container. Replace clippers or scissors that have become dull.

Orange stick or nail stone (made of a pumicelike substance) may be used to push back the cuticle gently. To prevent injury from using an orange stick, cover the stick with clean cotton before each use. Replace orange sticks that are frayed or worn down. Nail stones tend to be gentler than orange sticks and don't need to be replaced as frequently. Do *not* use metal cuticle trimmers or scissors. While a professional manicurist often uses them on clients, dermatologists say that most women don't have the expertise needed to use them properly on themselves. Cuticles can be cut back too far or unevenly, making the nails look unattractive and increasing the risks of infection.

Emery boards are generally the least expensive, most effective tools for filing nails. Use the rough side only if you want to file down much of your nail, the soft side for finishing touches or for light filing. Some manicurists recommend rubbing two emery boards together to "season" them, prevent them from being too abrasive at first. Metal nail files are generally not recommended because they are more likely to lead to broken and split nails.

Nail buffers can give a sheen of polish to bare nails and are great if you prefer to go without nail enamel or if you want a finished look to your nails without taking too much time. Look for fine buffers, especially those covered with suede or chamois cloth. Replace these when the fabric wears and the buffer doesn't produce as high a shine on the nails.

How to Manicure Your Fingernails

1. Stroke a cotton ball soaked in nail polish remover over the length of your entire nail in rapid movements until all the old nail polish is removed. (If your nails are very soft, leave the polish on until after you have filed your nails. By providing an extra layer of material, the polish makes your nails a bit stronger, less likely to break during filing.) Nail polish removers that come in jars in which you can dip your fingers may be convenient, but they expose more of your skin to the harsh chemicals in the remover unnecessarily. It is best to avoid them if possible.

2. Soak your fingertips in soapy water, cleaning the nails and cuticles thoroughly (but don't be rough).

3. File your nails using the smooth side of an emery board. Hold the emery board at a 45-degree angle to the nail. File in one direction—either up or down but not back and forth. Follow the natural shape of the nails; do not file in too closely on the sides of the nail or too straight across the top, which increases the chance of breakage. Many manicurists now say that the most practical and also most attractive length for nails is no longer than one-quarter inch beyond the fingertip.

4. Dip your fingertips in warm soapy water for one minute or so. Dry your hands and apply cuticle cream to soften the skin around your nails. If you want, you can use a damp facecloth to push back your cuticles gently at this point. Do not attempt to trim your cuticles or to push them back with a metal instrument; you will only raise your risk of injury and infection. There is no medical reason for cuticles to be trimmed; in fact, cuticles protect the nail, and so nails are healthiest when the cuticle is left intact. If you use cuticle cream, don't let the product

stay on your fingers longer than recommended in the instructions on the label; these products contain sodium hydroxide or calcium hydroxide, both of which can damage skin if left on for too long.

5. Rinse your hands in cool water to remove the cuticle cream and cuticle residue. Dry them gently.

6. Apply a clear base coat to nails first and wait for it to dry. Follow with two coats of colored enamel and one clear top coat. Allow ten minutes between coats for the enamel to dry.

7. Massage hand cream into your fingertips after the polish has dried completely.

8. To stretch the longevity of a manicure, reapply the top coat the day after the manicure and every other day until it's time for a new manicure. Wear cotton-lined plastic gloves when doing any housework and gardening gloves when working outside to protect nails.

Your Best Feet Forward: Ten Steps to a Perfect Pedicure

Because feet are covered up all day long and the toenails aren't exposed to the banging and chipping hazards of fingernails, a pedicure can last significantly longer (up to eight weeks) than a manicure. That's the good news. The bad news is that a pedicure also takes longer to do—bad news, that is, unless you love to pamper yourself.

1. Begin by removing any old polish on your toenails with a cotton ball soaked in nail polish remover.

2. Next, give your feet a luxurious soak in warm soapy water. Soak for ten to twenty minutes and then dry your feet by rubbing gently with a towel.

3. Use a pumice stone or callus remover to rub away calluses from around the toes and heels. Using an exfoliating scrub might also help to smooth the skin on your feet.

4. Dip your feet in water again to remove the residue from exfoliation and dry gently.

5. If desired, push the cuticles back with a damp wash-cloth. (Again, this is not necessary, but many women like to do it.)

6. Using a toenail clipper, trim the nails straight across. Do not shape them as you do your fingernails, as this can lead easily to ingrown toenails. Toenails should just skirt beyond the tip of the toe—not so short that they cut into the skin of the toe but not so long that they rip your hosiery or can be injured easily.

7. File the nails straight across with an emery board—just to remove nail straggles, not to shape them.

8. Place cotton balls between the toes to keep them from rubbing against each other and smudging the polish. Apply a base coat, one or two coats of nail polish, and a top coat to the nails, waiting ten minutes between coats to allow for adequate drying.

9. When the polish has dried completely (allow a good half hour), apply a rich moisturizer to your feet, followed by a pair of cotton socks.

10. To keep the skin on your feet smooth and soft, use a pumice stone to remove dry rough skin when you bathe or shower, and apply a rich moisturizing cream to your feet nightly or daily after showering and before putting on socks.

The New Fake Fingernails

The term *fake fingernails* used to refer most often to plastic nails that you bought in different sizes and glued onto your own nail for a big evening out or other occasion. They usually didn't stay on your fingers for more than a day or two and so were considered relatively harmless. Today artificial nails, sculpted nails, nail-mending materials, and nail wraps are made of materials ranging from paper, silk, and linen to fiberglass. They look much more natural than the fake fingernails of yesterday, and some are meant to last for several weeks at a time—a convenience that can mean trouble for the health of your nails. Water can get trapped between your natural nail and the fake extension above, creating the perfect environment for microorganisms to flourish, leading to fungal, yeast, or bacterial infections of the nail area. Sometimes these infections clear up readily when the nail is removed. Other times permanent damage to the nail may result. Some women may also develop allergic reactions to the glues used in artificial nails.

The best advice is to avoid the use of artificial nails altogether. But if you must use them, here are some guidelines for minimizing your risks.

- Choose the type of nail carefully. Generally, the less permanent the nails are, the safer they are too. Preglued "press-on" nails are the least likely to cause problems but should be removed within a day or so of application. (They should be avoided by women who have known allergies to acrylic adhesives.) Preformed nails that require the use of glue are the next least likely to injure your nails, but steer clear of them if you have been known to be allergic to glues in the past. Sculpted nails are least problematic when made of paper (about the thickness of teabag paper). Those made of acrylics may cause allergic reactions in sensitive women. Silk and linen wraps tend to be more occlusive and therefore hold in water more readily.

- Ask your manicurist about the feasibility of applying an antifungal medication to your fingernails before applying the false nails on top. Sometimes these products can prevent fungal infections from occurring.

- Never apply false fingernails to nails that already have fungal, yeast, or bacterial infections.

- Remove the nail at the first sign of trouble—redness, itching, pain.

- Sculpted nails should be replaced every three weeks, according to some dermatologists, or else the seal between the artificial nail and the natural nail will weaken, allowing moisture to get trapped between them and infection to ensue.

- Avoid accidental scratches caused by artificial nails. There have been reports in medical journals of women who have given themselves corneal ulcers because they scratched their eyes, having temporarily forgotten how much longer their artificial nails were than their natural nails. Be cautious!

- Realize that once a fake fingernail is glued to your nail, it may be hard to remove. There have been anecdotal reports of women whose own nails have been torn off when the fake nail got caught on strong objects. Fake fingernails may not be a safe option for you if you do a lot of rugged work with your hands.

Safety at the Nail Salon

A proper manicure involves the use of sharp instruments to cut away excess cuticle and to file and clean nails. Although accidents at a salon are not common, they can occur, and that means that the possibility of spreading infection is very real. The Centers for Disease Control and Prevention report that no case of hepatitis B or AIDS has ever been spread through patrons at a nail salon. That's the good news. The bad news is that spread of infections such as warts, fungal infections, and herpes simplex can occur fairly easily.

One way to minimize the risks of infection is to bring your own manicure utensils to a salon for a manicure. Most salons won't mind your doing so. At a recent meeting of the American Academy of Dermatology, Marianne O'Donoghue, M.D., associate professor of dermatology at Rush-Presbyterian/St. Luke's Medical School in Chicago, recommended looking for some of the following features to ensure that your visit to the nail salon is sanitary and safe.

- Check to see if your state licenses nail salons; if it does, make sure the salon you visit is licensed.

- See if the salon has a sign with a logo bearing the phrase "We Care" hanging in the window. These signs are given out by the National Nail Technicians Group (NNTG) to salons that have proven that they follow proper procedures for sanitation and safety.

- Ask how the salon sterilizes its manicuring utensils. The best method of sterilizing instruments is with heat, and it should be done between every patron, not just once a day. Rubbing alcohol is also effective at keeping instruments clean; some salons dip instruments into alcohol between use on each finger, not just each person, and this is best.

- Make sure your manicurist washes her hands before working on yours and asks that you wash yours too.

- Make sure you are given a fresh clean towel to use.

- Notice how the salon surfaces are sterilized. The salon workers should use bleach to clean countertops and basins for soaking feet (for pedicures). Formaldehyde is sometimes used but can cause problems for women who are sensitive to it.

- When fingernails are soaked, they should be put in fresh soapy water, not in warm hand lotion, which can spread infection. When hand lotion is applied, it should be dispensed from a pump bottle or a tube, not from a jar into which the manicurist dips her fingers.

CHAPTER 14

Drugstore Survival Guide for Your Nails

Americans spend more than $200 million on nail care annually, and every time you turn around, it seems that there are new products on the market, from basic polishes to hardeners, strengtheners, cuticle creams and conditioners, and assorted removers. Just how many products do you really need to keep your nails looking good? And what are the differences among all of them? Here is some clarification.

Nail Enamels

Anything that is applied as a "coat" to your nails is likely to have four basic ingredients:

1. A film former (usually nitrocellulose). As its name suggests, this ingredient helps the product to form a film that will adhere to your nail.
2. A thermoplastic resin (usually formaldehyde). This adds strength and gloss to the product and aids in adhesion to the nail.
3. A plasticizer (such as dibutyl phthalate and camphor). This ingredient gives the product some flexibility as it dries and prevents it from shrinking up on the nail.
4. One or more solvents, ingredients such as toluene, butyl and ethyl acetates, and isopropyl alcohol. Solvents make up about 75 percent of nail enamel products and

are used to keep the other ingredients in suspension and help the product flow smoothly out of the bottle. (The reason you need to shake nail polish before you apply it is to remix all the ingredients with the solvent for even coverage and color.)

In addition, if the nail enamel is colored, it will contain titanium dioxide or iron oxide. Pearlized or frosted nail polishes often contain guanine, an ingredient derived from fish scales that improves the light-reflecting qualities of the polish.

Most women can apply nail enamels without any consequences greater than occasional chipped color or a missed spot. But some women become sensitized to these ingredients, most commonly to formaldehyde, and allergic or irritant reactions can result. In many women the reaction shows up not on the hands, but in the eye area; this is because the skin in the eye area is the thinnest in the body and is therefore naturally more sensitive than the skin of the hands. Rubbing your eyes with freshly manicured fingertips may be enough to cause a reaction. In most cases just stopping use of the product enables the reaction to clear up on its own and prevents similar reactions in the future. The solvents in nail enamels probably won't cause allergies, but they can be dehydrating or irritating to nails and the skin around them. For this reason it's best to limit application of nail enamel to once a week or less.

Nail Polish Remover

Nail polish removers are designed to dissolve the hard film formed by nail enamels. Until a few years ago most nail polish removers contained acetone, a substance that works well to remove nail enamel but can be highly irritating to the skin around the nails and dehydrating to the nails themselves. Now more gentle removers are available that contain acetates; they work as well at removing the polish but tend to be less irritating and drying. Many so-called instant removers, in which women dip their fingers into a hole in the center of a sponge saturated with remover, still contain acetone, which can be especially harmful in this form because more of the skin is exposed to the remover than if the product were just wiped on with a cotton ball. If you've experienced irritation to removers in the past, avoid this type.

Most removers also contain alcohol and water, hydrolyzed animal proteins, and sometimes fragrance and artificial colors. If your skin tends to be irritated easily, it's best too look for a fragrance-free, clear formulation.

Nail Hardeners

Nail hardeners work by adding a strengthening layer to the nail, helping to prevent splitting and chipping. They contain the same four basic building blocks as nail enamel but also two other ingredients: formalin (or formaldehyde) and hydrolyzed protein. Protein generally does not cause irritation, but formaldehyde is a common allergen and sensitizer. For this reason some cosmetic companies offer nail hardeners with nonformaldehyde formulations. They don't harden as well as the formaldehyde-containing products, but they also are unlikely to cause irritation and so are best for women with very sensitive skin.

Some hardeners and strengtheners also contain tiny fibers, such as silk fibers, which can help form a tighter bond on the nail and resist peeling of the enamel. These products tend to be more resistant to removers, however, so they may not be the best choice for women who have had reactions to removers.

Cuticle Removers and Softeners

The active ingredient in cuticle removers is either sodium hydroxide or potassium hydroxide (types of lye). These actually help to dissolve the cuticle, making it easier to cut away or push back. Of course, since cuticles protect the nail, many doctors feel that use of these products is completely unnecessary and that they may be harmful if left on the skin for too long; skin swelling and redness may result from excess exposure to them. It's important to follow directions for use carefully.

Cuticle softeners often contain salicylic acid, urea, and/or lactic acid. They are gentler than cuticle removers, but in women who have sensitive skin they may cause chronic redness and inflammation and should be avoided if they produce this reaction.

Just how many coats of polish do your nails need? Probably not as many as you think. Generally, professional nail technicians recommend applying a base coat, two coats of enamel (one may be enough for very dark shades), and one top coat; many manicurists suggest reapplying a top coat every other day after the manicure to stretch the results and make the nail enamel more resistant to chipping and splitting. Since there's not much difference in formulation between base coats and top coats (just different percentages of the same ingredients), you can probably use them interchangeably without any problem. Clear nail hardeners may also be used as a base or top coat.

In recent years the look of "clean" nails—those that are rounded only about one-quarter inch over the fingertip and covered with a sheer or clear coat of polish—have come into fashion. These nails not only look professional and neat but are also easier to maintain and don't require an arsenal of products to achieve. Sometimes the simplest approach is, indeed, the best.

Index

Plantar warts, 64
Plaque psoriasis, 52–53
Pluckers, electric, 154–155
Plucking and tweezing hair, 154–155
Poison ivy, oak, and sumac, allergies to, 57
Polymer bases, 168
Pomade acne, 44, 138
Pomades, 138
Pores, 41
Port-wine stains, 10–11
Precancerous lesions, 81
Prednisone, 50
Pregnancy
    Accutane discontinued during, 49
    hair coloring avoided during, 132–133
    hair during, 120
    mask of, 75
    nails during, 179
    skin and, 17–18
Prescription medications
    for acne, 47–51
    sunlight and, 37
Preservatives in shampoos, 161
"Press-on" nails, 195
Prickly heat, 9
Progesterone, 16
Progressive hair color, 124
Pseudomonas, 71
Psoralen, 54, 59
    plus exposure to UVA (PUVA therapy), 74
Psoriasis, 52–54, 148–149
Puberty, 14, 40
Pucker lines, 19
Pumice stone, 193, 194
Purpura, 18
Pustules, 43
PUVA therapy (psoralen drugs plus exposure to UVA), 74
Pyruvic acid, 87

Radiation, 31
Rashes, 9
Razor bumps, 70
Razors, 152–153
Relaxers, chemical, for hair, 139–140
Renova, 85–86
Reproductive years
    hair in, 120–121
    nails in, 179
    skin in, 16–18
Resorcinol, 46–47, 82
Retinoic acid (Retin-A), 15, 37, 48–49, 82, 85–86

Reye's syndrome, 63
Rhinophyma, 77
Ringworm, 67–68
Rinsing hair, 165
Rinsing skin, 109
Rogaine, 145–146
Rosacea, 77–78
Rubella (German measles), 13–14

Salicylic acid, 46–47
Scalp problems, 147–149
Scaly skin, 9
Scars, 7
Sclerosing solutions, 79
Sebaceous glands, 14, 41
Seborrhea, 148
Seborrheic dermatitis, 117, 148, 149
Seborrheic keratoses, 20–21
Sebum (oil), 41
Selenium sulfide, 69
Self-exam, skin, 29–30
Self-starvation (anorexia), 15, 178
Self-tanning products, 37–39
Semi-permanent hair color, 124–125
Sensitive skin, 8
Sex hormones, 14
Shampoo-and-conditioner-in-one products, 164
Shampoos, 159
    choosing and using, 159–164
    for different types of hair, 163–164
    ingredients in, 160–163
    switching, 165
Shaving, 151–153
Shedding skin cells, 5
Shingles, 60, 64
Silicone, 87
Skiing, 7
Skin, 3
    with acne, 41
    acne-prone, see Acne-prone skin
    in adolescence, 14–16
    aging, 18–21
    anatomy of, 4–7
    antiaging, 81–89
    black, 20
    chemical peels for, 81–84
    in childhood, 12–14
    cleansing, 15
    dry, 7–8
    in fifty-plus, 18–21
    in infancy, 8–12
    oily, 7–8
    pale, 15
    peeling, 5

About the Author

Laura Flynn McCarthy spent six years on the staff of *Vogue* Magazine as a writer and editor, first in the features department, and then in the health and beauty department. Since becoming a freelance writer in 1988, she has written for more than twenty-five different magazines including *Cosmopolitan, Harper's Bazaar, McCall's, Fitness, Self, Mademoiselle, Working Woman* and *Seventeen*. She has won two awards for excellence in science writing. She lives in New Hampshire with her husband and their son.